# IRISH FOLK CURES

### Padraic O'Farrell

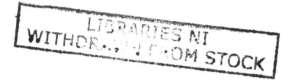

Gill & Macmillan

*Gill & Macmillan Ltd*
*Hume Avenue, Park West, Dublin 12*
*with associated companies throughout the world*
*www.gillmacmillan.ie*
© *The Estate of the late Padraic O'Farrell 2004*
*0 7171 3617 5*
*Original text design by*
*Identikit Design Consultants, Dublin*
*Print origination by Carole Lynch*
*Printed and bound by Nørhaven Paperback A/S, Denmark*

*This book is typeset in 10/15 pt Adobe Garamond.*

The paper used in this book comes from the wood pulp
of managed forests. For every tree felled, at least one tree
is planted, thereby renewing natural resources.

*A CIP catalogue record for this book is available*
*from the British Library.*

# CONTENTS

# INTRODUCTION

Flavius Josephus commanded a Galilean force during the Jewish revolt against Rome in 66 AD. He produced several works of history and was said to have claimed that the Irish alone preserved secrets of the mystic power of herbs to instil hate and love and to cure illness. They knew of an unnamed 'fairy plant' and how to use it to gain power over beings of the Otherworld – fairies and demons.

Irish bards knew of a potion that, given to a newborn child, could bestow a sweet singing voice, which in adulthood could make a listener, who was ill, forget pain and be soothed into a pleasant sleep. Fionn Mac Cumhaill's court bard at the Hill of Allen in County Kildare was an example.

The attribution of healing to supernatural powers originated long before the establishment of modern medicine in the seventeenth century. It was a universal phenomenon. Native American chiefs, African witch doctors, and medical men in Australia, Europe and Asia, all held the respect of their communities. In Ireland people were simply unaware of any possible source of illness other than a hostile spirit. There was a strong tradition of fairy lore and a deeply religious ethos among the Irish, and belief in both often clashed. 'Superstitious observances of omens and actions are very sinful,' preached the priest. 'God is good but don't dance in a *naomhóg* [currach, coracle],' said the pragmatist, and so he tried in every way to cure his illness.

Modern living has altered society and sophisticated lifestyles make people poor subjects for deriving any benefit from Irish folk cures. Also, it must be said that many of the cures in this book appear quite outlandish and perhaps should be taken with a pinch of salt – or dandelion seed, or crushed hemlock or ash of burnt mice!

## ABOUT THE BOOK'S TERMS AND STRUCTURE

To avoid repetition, in most cases I use the term 'healer' for convenience when I refer to an unqualified 'doctor', 'wise man' or 'wise woman'. And flying in the face of Biddy Early and her feminist descendants, I use the pronoun 'he' for convenience. Mainly, I use the past tense but in supplying recipes or treatments in list form without elaboration, the present tense is used. For brevity and conciseness, I avoid stating that people believed in the cures and in their outcome. I simply refer to treatments as if they were positive remedies.

## WARNING

The cures cited in this book have not been scientifically validated nor is their use recommended. Some are positively dangerous – the use of arsenic or caustic soda, in particular. There has been at least one case of a man who used an arsenic plaster on a wart losing his finger.

This book, therefore, comes with a publisher's and author's warning. No responsibility is accepted for those who experiment. After all, modern living has deprived people of the 'knack' in the use of folk cures.

**Padraic O'Farrell, 2003**


PUBLISHER'S NOTE
Padraic O'Farrell died suddenly while this book was in preparation. He was, in the most literal sense, an officer and a gentleman. He had served with distinction as a colonel in the Irish army. His love of literature and drama was a constant in his life. On his retirement, he was able to dedicate himself fully to these pursuits. He was a prolific and punctilious author and a delightful companion. He died shortly after reading and approving the proofs of this book. He left everything just so, in good order, and is much missed.

ONE

# ANIMALS

Irish country people had great affection for
animals, whether wild, livestock or pets, and
they held some wild animals in awe. The hare, for
example, featured in *piseóga* as some unfortunate
human under a spell. Cows and their produce were
associated with all sorts of customs and
superstitions, and fairies seem to have had a
particular fondness for interfering with milk yields.
Irish folk cures, therefore, concerned animals as
well as humans, and no self-respecting healer
specialising in, say, bone fractures, would have
survived in his calling if he were not able to apply
his skills to a horse's dodgy fetlock as well as a fair
lady's ankle. The person who could make a sick
beast well won widespread respect. If he attended
to beasts alone, he won the appellation 'cow
doctor'. His amulets and 'tools of the trade' were
cherished possessions. A court case in Cork in
1840 involved the robbery of a stone that could
cure any disease in a cow by rubbing it on the
beast's back. It was claimed that the fairies had
given it to MacCarthy Mór, an ancient King of
Munster, and it had been handed down through
generations. The judge wryly stated that the matter
was outside his jurisdiction, but the plaintiff, a Mrs
McAuliffe, vowed that the alleged robber's family,

the Sheehans, would thaw away like ice in the sun. Today, however, if you throw a stone in Cork you will hit a Sheehan!

From the fourteenth to the seventeenth century, Cassidys were physicians to the Maguire chieftains in County Fermanagh. Thereafter, families named Cassidy kept a 'Cassidy's Rag' torn from any old garment. By placing it in any beast's drinking water, it could cure almost any ailment.

There are theories that many precious manuscripts were destroyed by 'cow doctors'. Part of their technique involved dipping them in water, which they then used for healing. They also used relics, chalices and bells, and wax from church candles.

Livestock farmers had faith in Saint Blaise and believed that praying to him, especially on his feast day, 2 February, could cure ailing cattle. (For other cures associated with the feast day of Saint Blaise, *see* Throat.) For undiagnosed illnesses, they squeezed nine leaves of crowfoot picked on a Sunday night against a newly unearthed rock. After spitting on it, they added salt and smeared the animal's ear with the paste.

CATTLE

Superstitions concerning the care of cows and their milk was widespread. Rituals for their protection were common. One of Ireland's most famous cows was Glas Ghaibhne (Grey Cow of Gabhne). It was a magic beast belonging to Cian, son of Dian Cécht, the god of medicine. Balor of the Evil Eye stole it and brought it to Tory Island. Cian went there and recovered it, but not before he seduced Balor's daughter.

### Abortion
Place a goat among the herd.

### Anthrax
Hang the placenta of a cow or mare on a hawthorn bush. Leave there until it disintegrates or is decimated by birds of prey. This protects the livestock from anthrax and similar diseases.

*See also* Blood Disorders.

### Blackleg (Black Quarter)
An early practice equating to primitive inoculation took place in some farming communities. If a calf died of 'black quarter', the affected leg was cut off and hung in the chimney as a charm against the disease. In more remote areas, however, it was left only until cured like bacon. Then the farmer pulverised it and spread it on a narrow tape. Using a jute needle, he pressed this as a seton into a fold above a young calf's hip.

**Other treatments:**
- Cut the flesh and insert a clove of garlic. Stitch or bandage.

- Tie a circle of loose red thread through the cow's dewlap.

### Bloat

Gasses building up in the stomach cause this swelling. The farmer allowed them to escape by sticking a narrow knitting needle into the stomach.

**Other treatments:**

- Mix one teaspoonful each of pulverised gentian blossom, ginger, bread soda and ammonia with two teaspoonfuls of charred alder wood. Mix into the animal's feed.

### Calving

After having her first calf, the farmer lit a blessed candle and passed it backwards and forwards between the heifer's hind legs. Then, with its flame, he burned off the hair around the udder. This encouraged a good milk yield. After subsequent calving, he first passed the lit candle over the beast's back, under the stomach and finally between the hind legs.

### Diarrhoea

*See* Scour, *below.*

### Elf Shoot

If a cow's milk yield lessened suddenly, its owner normally blamed fairy stroke or elf shoot, caused by fairies firing darts. Using lengths from his elbow to fingertips, the 'cow doctor' measured the beast from the root of the tail to the top of the head and then the opposite way. Somehow, disparity between the measurements was not unknown and was a sign of the fairy stroke. The cure was to force the cow to drink some water from a mearing ditch or stream between parishes.

**Other treatments:**

• Measure the beast's girth three times. Locate the mark left by the dart. Rub with an elf-stone (usually a Stone Age arrowhead).

### Farcy

*See* Horses, *below*.

Some of the cures for warts in humans (*see* Warts, *under* Skin) were administered for farcy in cattle.

### Milk

Every dairyman squirted the first drop on his finger, made the Sign of the Cross on the cow's flank and said, 'God bless the cow!' A cup was kept in the stable and if a visitor called, he was offered (and was expected to accept) a small drop of milk to drink, after which he would say, 'God bless the cows!' All this helped keep the fairies at bay.

Fairy interference with milk is a regular feature of folklore (see my *Irish Customs* in this Gill & Macmillan series). A County Carlow farmer was finding that from the milk of seven cows his wife was only getting froth when she churned. Half a mile away, the milk from his farmhand's single cow was providing incredible amounts of butter. The farmer consulted Moll Anthony the wise woman of County Kildare and followed her advice during his wife's next churning.

After giving his farmhand a job to do in a distant field, he heated the coulter of his plough until red hot and plunged it into the milk. Then he wrapped the plough chains around the churn. He locked the door and told his wife to begin. Immediately, the farmhand rushed from the field in agony. His stomach was burning inside and he screamed in pain. He ran to the house and began hammering on the door, begging for admission. The farmer pitied him but knew he must stick to Moll's advice. The churning produced a normal amount of butter and the farmhand's pain left him. At his next churning, however, his cow's yield too was back to normal.

### Milk Fever

Over-production of milk, particularly after calving, caused this serious ailment. After milking, the farmer pumped air into each teat with a bicycle pump and valve until the udder was inflated. He then bound them tightly with bandages to keep the air in, so that milk could not form.

**Other treatments:**

- Mix lime into the cow's drinking trough.
- Pulverise hawthorn or buttercup blooms and store the juices in a sealed container. Rub on the udder when required.
- The cure for blasts in humans (*see* Skin) could also cure a swollen udder.

### *Murrain (Red Murrain, Red Water)*

Pilgrims to the Middle East were in the habit of bringing back crystals to Ireland and they were used in folk medicine. To cure murrain or distemper in cattle, Waterford farmers borrowed a crystal brought from the Holy Land that belonged to the le Poer family. They placed it in a stream through which they drove the cattle backwards and forwards a few times.

In Munster, farmers kept a dead 'conach worm' or 'conach moth' in the cow byre to protect the animals against this dreaded disease (*see* Donkeys, *below*).

**Other treatments:**

- Anoint with the blood of a Keogh.
- Feed the cow the contents of two bags of laundry blue.
- Mix treacle with mulled stout and give to drink.
- Mix salt in lard and give to eat.
- Give copious amounts of strong tea to drink.

d dye from the root of a pound of
...er into two gallons of human urine and
Pulverise the remainder of the madder
and stir the powder into a pound each of alum
and tar. Add to the boiling mixture and stir.
While dropping in clippings of straw from a
pallet, say the Lord's Prayer five times, and five
Hail Marys and the Apostles' Creed. When
cool, force the sick cow to drink a hornful.
Then mark a cross on the snout, over the right
eye and on the palate.

### Ringworm

Many of the cures used for humans applied (*see*
Children).

**Other treatments:**

- Clean with paraffin oil (kerosene) and then
  apply archangel tar or iodine.

### Scour

- Feed calves with bulbs of an umbellifer known
  as wild parsley.
- Chop and boil comfrey leaves. Mix into the
  animal's feed.

### Sore Eyes

A farmer's wife always kept an ivy leaf hanging over
the chimney. As the leaf dried, all soreness from
cows' eyes disappeared.

**Other treatments:**

- Mix lime in water and bathe the eyes.

### Sores

Some of the cures for humans applied (*see* Sores, *under* Skin).

**Other treatments:**

- Pulverise bluestone. Mix with rendered beef suet. Use as ointment.

### Sterility

Place a goat among the herd.

### Warble Fly Swelling

Clip hair around swelling. Cut a wound. Clean out infection and disinfect. Dress with white of egg.

### Warts

Most of the methods used with humans applied to cattle (*see* Warts, *under* Skin).

### Worms

**Tail worm ('Worm in the tail'):** The 'cow doctor' uttered incantations before making an incision in the tail close to where it met the back. He stuffed this with a mixture of turpentine, rue and garlic before binding it with a red cloth.

**Worm attack (*Ruathar péisteanna*):** This ailment called for a strange treatment. With his own hat or cap, a 'cow doctor' tapped the animal on its back, then tied a string (*rucrapeist*) across its back with a knot that opened when each end of the string was pulled. He did this three times, uttering a secret prayer each time. Worms, colic or gripe were 'caught' in the knot and 'fell' to the end of the string and away. Some communities called the practice *sníomh na péiste* (worm or reptile's twist).

**Other treatments:**

* Grind down a sod of turf. Add salt and soot. Dampen into a paste and give to the cow to eat.

## DOGS

Because the dog is 'man's faithful friend', it is a popular pet, but on the land, especially among mountain sheep farmers, it is an indispensable aid to stock management. Watching a well-trained sheep dog going about its work on a mountainside is fascinating. Happily for their masters, dogs did not suffer from many maladies.

### Distemper

Mix sulphur in milk and give to drink.

### Mange

Mix four ounces of sulphur with one ounce of mercury ointment, one of turpentine and half an ounce of tar spirit. Mix into a pint of linseed oil. Rub on affected parts.

### Rabies

Afflicted animals were brought to sit on the

Madman's Chair in Dunany Point, near
Clogherhead, County Louth (*see* Mental Ailments).

### Ringworm
Apply seaweed or iodine to affected parts. Some of
the treatments for humans applied (*see* Children).

DONKEYS
There was a subdued respect for the animal that
carried the Virgin to Bethlehem to give birth to
Jesus and later bore the adult Jesus into Jerusalem.

Handy about the farm, the donkey was also the
only animal able to kill the 'conach worm' (or moth),
which caused murrain and other ailments. Farmers
placed a hair from the cross of its back on a wound
and any worm or moth alighting near it died.

### Dung Eating
Donkeys have a habit of eating dung, which can
lead to internal infections. To discourage the
practice, mix red pepper or eggshells into dung in
the animal's vicinity.

### Strangle(s)
An infectious, chain-forming bacteria causes a fever
accompanied by coughing (also in horses); its
common name is strangles. Crush primrose roots.
Strain. Mix with whey of goat's milk. Press into the
nostrils frequently.

## HORSES

Hack, hunter, plough-horse or racehorse – the Irish have a high regard for horses. The animal appears in mythology and in folklore, and its finest hour was before the advent of the tractor, when the horse pulled cart and plough and carried his master around his holding. So the animal's health was vital to the running of a farm and folk cures were common.

### Back

A plaster of belladonna or mustard strengthened weak back muscles.

### Bleeding

Feed with curly kale or green cabbage leaves. Dress with the *cáise Púca* (cosha Pooka).

*See also* Wounds, *under* Blood.

### Bots

This is a disease caused by the parasitic maggot of the botfly. It normally enters the horse's stomach when the beast licks a wound infected by it.

Give the animal a gallon of sweetened milk to drink. Turn him on his back. The bots will fall into the milk and will eventually be passed out.

### Broken Wind

A spasm of the larynx sometimes presents a horse with breathing problems. Line the bottom of the horse's drinking trough with archangel tar. If the horse refuses the water because of the taste, keep him thirsty until he drinks it.

**Other treatments:**

- Give the horse the whites of twelve eggs each morning.

### Chafing (Gall)

Dabbing with salted water, human urine or whiskey can prevent or alleviate light chafing from harness. If proud (overgrown) flesh forms, cut away and apply a plaster of salted egg yolk. Leave until it falls off, then wash in urine for four days.

**Other treatments:**

- Apply a mixture of tar and fuller's earth.

### Colic

Dose with laudanum and allow to sleep in fresh straw.

### Congestion

Sear the horse's palate with a red-hot iron.

### Coughing

Apply a mustard blister pack to the lower jaw.

### Cuts and Grazes

If there is pus, cauterise. Make a plaster of butter, egg yolk and sheep's dung. Apply for three days. Then apply a further plaster of rendered sheep suet, butter, pulverised dock, chickweed and boiled marsh mallow.

**Other treatments:**
- Apply a plaster of pulverised elm bark mixed with rendered sheep suet.

## Farcy

Place a poultice of dried mud from the bottom of a lake or bog around the swelling (in some areas, the leg is first cut and two pints of blood removed). Fast the animal for twenty-four hours, then force him to drink a mixture of turpentine and linseed oil. This will cause vomiting. Then gallop him until he defecates. After a few days on grass, the horse will be cured.

## Frog Thrush

Thrush in the elastic horny substance in the middle of a horse's hoof (the frog) can cause lameness. It normally creates a crack into which roasted salt should be poured and kept in place with a rag. Hard frog, on the other hand, requires a dressing of linseed oil or cow dung.

## Itch

Pulverise dock roots, alum, clover and honeysuckle. Boil with lard and honey. Strain. Add sulphur and mix into an ointment. Apply to itchy hooves.

## Lampers (Mouth Blisters)

Mix gorse clippings in the animal's feed. These will burst the mouth blisters and the horse's natural instinct to lick the thorns away will cure less severe cases (a human can do the bursting, but must be careful).

### Sprains

Boil dock leaves in water and strain. Mix leaves in unsalted butter. Heat antiphlogistine and smear on brown paper. Apply to sprained area and bandage.

**Other treatments:**

- Massage with soap and water.

### Strangle(s)

*See* Donkey, *above.*

### Temper

A regular diet of wild parsley (sometimes called horse parsley) can tame an ill-tempered horse.

### Warts

Cut off and cauterise or squeeze with hot tongs. Some of the cures for humans apply.

*See* Warts, *under* Skin.

### Weeping Heels

Inadequate cleanliness in the stable can cause this complaint, which is also known as greasy heels. First, the stable must be thoroughly cleaned and disinfected. Then the ailment can be tackled. Remedies include application of archangel tar or bluestone. If the malady persists, apply a poultice of grated carrots for three consecutive days. Change the poultice to sodden bread for another three. If there is still no improvement, apply a poultice of human excrement.

### Worms

Pulverise the yellow blossom of gorse. Mix with linseed oil and give to the horse to eat. Some of the remedies for cattle (*above*) apply.

## PIGS

Irish mythology abounds in epic tales of chasing wild boars. At great banquets, pompous ceremony accompanied the carving of the beast. Some enchanted boars reappeared even after being killed and eaten. The common domestic pig, however, does not appear often in folklore.

### General Health

Chop dandelion leaves and roots. Boil and add to feed.

### Scour

Place a fistful of flour and a spoonful of alum in milk and boil. Feed to the animal once each day until cured.

### Swine Fever

Chop roots of comfrey and boil in milk. Mix into feed for three weeks or until cured.

### Weak Legs
Add limewater and cod liver oil to the feed.

SHEEP

It is a pleasant experience to watch a shepherd and his dog rounding up sheep on a mountainside. Once, there was a custom whereby, if a shepherd died, his next-of-kin placed a fistful of sheep's wool in his coffin. This meant he would be excused for having missed Sunday Mass on days he was minding his flock. Sheep with heavy fleeces got hot and dirty and were prone to diseases.

### Foot Rot
Pare away soft horn and apply archangel tar.

### Liver Fluke
Mix the blooms of any yellow flower (iris, ragwort, buttercup, dandelion) and feed to the animal.
- Apply a compound of antimony butter externally around the liver area.

### Maggots
Shear wool from affected sore and use some to wipe away larvae. Wash with salted buttermilk.

TWO

# BACK PAIN

A floating stone guided Saint Declan in his voyage to Ireland (see my *Irish Saints* in this Gill & Macmillan series). The stone lies on the beach at Ardmore, County Waterford. On his feast day (24 July), back sufferers crawled beneath this stone for relief. A similar practice took place at Saint Rónán's Altar (or Mass Table) at Kilronan, near Ballyfarnan, County Roscommon. Patients also lay on Saint Columcille's Bed by his holy well near Inver, County Donegal, and on Saint Molaise's Bed on Devenish Island, Lough Erne, County Fermanagh.

**Other treatments:**

- Apply hot poultices of bog onion or garlic.
- Heat a brick and press it against the aching area.
- Fill a lidded earthenware vessel with boiling water and seal the lid. Lie in bed with the vessel against the back.
- Pulverise deadly nightshade (belladonna) and mix two teaspoonfuls of its juice to eight of olive oil. Add camphor oil, if available. Use as a liniment.
- Pulverise monkshood and add three teaspoonfuls of its juice to two of lard. Massage the affected area.

THREE

# BLOOD DISORDERS

Michael Forde of Tullynaha, County Cavan, had an instrument called a 'flame' for extracting blood from a patient. He allowed about a pint of blood to flow into a dish, where froth would appear on it if it contained impurities. Treatments varied. By the seaside, both healers and householders knew of a variety of seaweed, found on the seabed, that had healing properties. It was collected at low tide, scraped and cut into strips, which were boiled in milk. This drinking potion cleansed the blood, and was especially effective for patients suffering from boils, pimples, rashes or other dermal complaints.

Drinking the juice of boiled nettles, bogbean, carrots or soot mixed in water also purified the blood. Three cupfuls on each of the first three days of May were particularly effective. In some areas boiled whitethorn blooms were substituted. Three meals of nothing else but boiled nettles in one day each spring and regular doses of sulphur mixed in treacle were also popular treatments.

**Other treatments:**
- Chew the red seaweed, dulse (*dileasg*).
- Drink tansy or dock tea.
- Eat raw or boiled dandelion leaves.

- Boil a mixture of wood sorrel, dandelions and nettles. Cool and drink a pint daily.

## ABSCESS

Boil one parsnip. Remove and mash. Use the water in which it was boiled to bathe the abscess. Apply the mashed parsnip as a poultice. When soft, heat a needle and pierce the tip. Discontinue poultice but bathe regularly with warm water or warm vinegar. Ensure regular bowel movement.

## ANAEMIA

Pulverise wood sorrel, dandelions and nettles. Boil in the water from a 'brown' stream (i.e. with iron content in its water). Cool and drink a pint daily.

## ANTHRAX (QUARTER EVIL; TANNER'S DISEASE)

Anthrax can result from working with cattle. Swab ulcers with red flannel dipped in carbolic acid. Apply any hot poultice.

## BLEEDING NOSE

- Place a key or some cold object (e.g. a spoon) on the patient's back, inside the clothing.
- Place a cold stone or metal object against the forehead.
- Press the nostrils together but do not swallow the blood.

## BLOOD PRESSURE

The patient sits. A healer moves his hands upward from the toes to the head but never touches any part of the body. He prays silently. He then sprinkles water on the legs. This occurs during three visits at regular intervals.

About fourteen years ago, my wife and I were suffering from very high blood pressure. She visited the late Michael Cully of Derrinturn, Carbury, County Kildare, and received treatment similar to that outlined above. She had faith in him and advised me to accompany her when she was going for her second visit. 'Even if you do not believe in his ability to cure, you will like him and he will help your research into folklore,' Maureen suggested. She was right. He was a gentle man and I felt that if God did choose people to cure the sick, it would surely be a man like this. Although still dubious, I made the three visits. After the third, I asked Michael what I should do about the medication I was taking for blood pressure. He told me to consult my doctor.

I went to see my doctor and my wife visited hers. Although she was a firm believer in the healer, her blood pressure was still high and she has remained on medication ever since. Mine, on the other hand, was normal and remained so for a number of years. Although it rose occasionally during the past decade, I have not been on medication until recently. Injustices occur in folk medicine too.

## DIABETES
Ingest cranesbill (*crobh dearg*) by any method.

## INTERNAL BLEEDING
Boil plantain (*slánlus*) in water and drink while hot.

## JAUNDICE
The 'yellow ganders' (or jaunders) was the name for jaundice (*liath buidhe*), whether it was of the black or yellow type. Wild yellow blooms formed the basis of a number of remedies. The patient drank the water in which mustard (charlock), ragwort, yellow iris or buttercups had been boiled. Sometimes, the boiled plants were placed on the eyes and up the nostrils. Parents who had the same surname before marriage placed a donkey's halter on their jaundiced child and led it to a well. The child drank three times from it.

**Other treatments:**

- Tiny hairs on sundew, an insectivorous bog plant, secrete moisture. If the moisture is mixed in milk and boiled with some of the plant's leaves and drunk every day for a fortnight, a cure will follow.
- Every day for a fortnight, mix the patient's urine with the same amount of milk and give to the patient to drink.

- Pulverise one ounce each of ginger, camomile blossoms, dandelion roots and senna. Mix into boiling water. When cool, take a half teaspoonful twice daily.
- Eat soup made from snails.
- Boil goats' droppings in fresh milk. Drink when cool.
- Boil goose excrement in milk. Drink when hot.
- Give a donkey some cake to eat. Gather the crumbs and give them to the patient to eat.
- Swallow up to a dozen live lice from a pig.
- Pulverise lice and mix in the patient's food.
- Take nine fresh shoots from the root of an ash tree. Place them in a bottle and bury in a spot where the patient will not find it. This will effect a cure, but if the bottle breaks or is found, the disease will return in a more chronic form.
- Boil saffron, marigold or lilac in milk left over after a ferret has drunk. Drink when cool.
- Drink water from a spa near Wexford town (*near Spa-Well Brewery on Griffiths' Valuation Map, 1840*).

## WOUNDS

'To rub salt on an open wound' is an expression used to describe the act of making someone's pain even worse. While salt in a wound is indeed painful, it nevertheless has healing properties and was used in folk medicine. A wide blade of grass could stem the flow of blood from a cut. Larger wounds called for a cobweb or for a tuft of fur pulled from a hare. A puffball fungus (*cáise Púca*) applied to the wound and held in place with a bandage, or its dust spread on the bandage, stemmed the flow also.

It was customary to kill a cock on Saint Martin's Day (11 November; *see* my *Irish Customs* in this Gill & Macmillan series). A cloth was soaked in its blood and kept in the rafters, and had the power to stop bleeding.

A stone beside a small waterfall near Lavey, County Cavan, always contained water in its two hollows. Kneeling in them cured wounds.

Moss, especially if collected from the walls of a church, features frequently in folk medicine and occasionally in history. Returning from the Battle of Clontarf in 1014, the armies of Desmond and Thomond camped at Magh Maistean, a plain near Athy. A long-standing dispute about the kingship of Munster, then held by Thomond, erupted. The Desmondites realised that Thomond casualties at Clontarf were considerable and that their King of Munster was wounded, so they demanded that a Desmond king be appointed to rule the province. Confrontation was inevitable. While both sides were preparing for action, the warriors from Thomond brought their wounded comrades to the Rath of Mullamast for safety. These men resented being left out of battle, however, and stuffed their wounds with moss before returning to join in the fray. Their bravery scared the men of Desmond into withdrawing from hostilities and continuing their march southward. There have been reports that sphagnum moss, soaked in garlic oil, was used as an antiseptic during the First World War, and was thought to have been one of the reasons for the low rate of infection among British soldiers compared with those of other armies.

**Other treatments:**

- Suck small cuts, then wash in clean water and apply friar's balsam.
- Soak bandages in the blood of twelve wrens. Bind the wound with one of them each day until it heals.
- Bathe in water that has washed a corpse.
- Bathe with soap and sugar.
- Bathe with human urine.
- Chew ribgrass or plantain and apply.
- Soak plantain in water. Apply.
- Apply pig dung.
- Boil a clove of garlic in milk and drink.
- Apply calf dung mixed with vinegar (also a cure for warts).
- Apply a poultice of human or cow's excrement.
- Apply a poultice of soot from a turf fire.
- Roast, then mash six potatoes. Add cream until it forms a thick paste. Apply as a poultice.

- Wash with carbolic soap.
- Boil plantain, marsh mallow, Jacob's ladder, foxglove or hemlock. Allow to cool, then drink the liquid.
- After chewing sorrel leaves, spit on the wound and rub on newly churned, unsalted butter.
- Crush yarrow, apply and bandage.
- Make an ointment from rendered beef suet and yarrow and apply.
- Chop groundsel and mix with oatmeal porridge. Dampen with hot water and use as a poultice.
- Take a burning sod of turf and scatter sugar on it. Hold the cut over it.
- Strap the wound with membrane from animal flesh.
- Strap a piece of raw meat to the wound.

FOUR

# BONES

A bonesetter employed some athletic methods of leverage. By lying on the floor alongside the patient and placing a foot under his armpit and pulling, he separated sections of a fractured shoulder. He might also sling a patient's broken arm over a half-door and tug it. Bandages soaked in soot or flour mixed with egg white acted as a light plaster. Scraps of sacking soaked in heated pitch and resin provided a stronger one. Bonesetters used primitive splints also.

'I can feel it in my bones' – imminent bad weather or 'a stepmother's bite in the wind' could cause pains and aches in the bones. While fractures were a matter for the bonesetter, sufferers of less serious but nagging complaints sought advice on temporary relief rather than cures. Some major ailments, however, required healers and home treatment.

## ARTHRITIS

Fairy darts caused red and inflamed joints associated with arthritis. A healer who could cure this complaint had to receive a request to do so; he could never offer his services unbidden. Among genuine healers there were a few fakes, like the person who produced the 'dart' from under the flesh and let it fall. The relatives of the patient then saw that it was only a sliver of straw made to appear that it had emerged from beneath the skin through sleight of hand.

**Treatments:**

- Remove the fairy dart that caused the arthritis by brushing the area with mint leaves or hemlock.
- Rub affected area(s) with a stolen potato.
- Rub affected area(s) with a cross-shaped bud taken from any tree in a cemetery.
- Slap the affected area with a holly sprig.

HIP BONE

In complete silence, find three green pebbles in the bed of a stream between midnight and dawn. Place each pebble on the hip and move it along the flesh as far as the big toe saying:

*Caith! Caith!*
*Fan as láthair*
*Pian cruálach.*
*Imigh! Imigh!*

*Wear away! Wear away!*
*Stay away*
*Cruel pain.*
*Away! Away!*

## JOINTS

In modern times it is customary to wear a copper
bracelet or carry crystals to alleviate joint pains. A
similar older version involved wearing an iron ring
on the fourth finger of the right hand.

**Swelling of joints:** Bandages or poultices of a
number of plants give relief. These include
hemlock, mountain sage, houseleek, comfrey root,
marsh mallow and cabbage leaves.

Mix one teaspoonful of sulphuric acid into
sixteen of olive oil. Allow to stand for fifteen
minutes and add a tablespoonful of turpentine. Use
as a liniment.

*See also* Arthritis, *above* and Back Pain.

## STIFF NECK

Massage and apply hot red flannel.

FIVE

# CANCER

There was once such despair about all forms of cancer that some healers advised the cure, *smut éadaigh a bheadg ar bhean chéile sagairt* (a rag of clothing that would be on a priest's wife – regarded then as an impossibility). There were other healers, however, who did offer remedies. One involved rolling a goose egg over the patient's body while mumbling a secret invocation.

## SKIN CANCER

- Make an ointment of butter or lard with arsenic, creosote, pitch or boiled ivy leaves. Place on a bandage and apply. Leave for nine days. When removed, it will take the growth (or part thereof) with it. Repeat if necessary, after a nine day rest.
- Rub dottle or ash from the bottom of a pipe on the growth.
- Apply water from a 'brown' river, i.e. a river with iron content in its waters.
- Wash with caustic soda.

SIX

# CHILDREN

In Ireland the adage 'Ne'er cast a clout till May is out' warned against forsaking even a patch (clout) of clothing until the blooming of the hawthorn (may). Yet, at the first sign of good weather parents decked their young daughters in pretty print dresses, their sons in light fabrics and allowed them to go barefoot to school and to play outdoors. The children delighted in the feel of dust on their feet as they scampered along unmetalled roads or caught buttercups and knapweed (blackheads) between their toes as they tripped through the fields.

People believed that a 'dawny' child – one fading away from no apparent illness – had received a fairy stroke. One remedy was the juice of twelve leaves of foxglove taken daily. Another was a series of visits to a stream in Culdaff, County Donegal, inaccurately called Saint Ultan's Well, preferably on the first Monday of January, April, July and October. At this place the mother did stations there on the child's behalf, crossing the stream, splashing its waters against a small waterfall above it, kissing a cross that stood there and saying prescribed prayers. She also took some of the water home and anointed the child with it daily. In more recent times, parents brought children suffering from bronchial problems to smell hot tar during road surfacing.

There were people who would never step over their child while it was playing on the kitchen floor. This, they feared, would stunt growth. A mother often pressed a child's wound together with her ring finger and thumb while saying:

> In the name of the Father and of the Son
> and of Holy Mary. The wound was deep,
> the blood was red and the flesh was
> painful but there will be no more blood or
> pain until Mary bears another child.

If a woman gave birth to a son on Good Friday, she usually asked that he be baptised with the newly blessed oils on Easter Sunday, something that would endow the child with the gift of healing.

## ASTHMA

- Chop and press leaves from the bog plant sundew. Mix with honey and fill into bottles. Keep some in stock always and take a tablespoonful when an attack occurs.
- Drink milk in which onions have been boiled.
- Keep vinegar in a saucer beside the child's bed.

## BED-WETTING

- Cook a mouse and pulverise it. Add it to some food the child likes. Feed to the child.

## CONVULSIONS

- Loosen the child's clothing. Sit it in a mustard bath for twenty minutes. If necessary, open the child's mouth with your fingers to aid breathing. Sponge the head with cold water. Dry well and put to bed.

- Boil foxglove in some water taken from a mearing stream where three holdings meet. When the signs of convulsions appear, have the child drink a cupful. Treat regularly with the concoction, even when the fits abate.

- Clip the child's nails and trim its hair. Wrap the clippings in linen and place them under the crib.

## COUGHS

- Pour boiling water into a narrow-topped, earthenware utensil. Mix in a half teaspoonful of friar's balsam. Keep the child's nose close to the top and allow it to inhale.

- Allow a half teaspoonful of warm olive oil to trickle down the child's throat every fifteen minutes.

- Rub chest, throat and between shoulder blades with warm olive oil.

- Soak two squares of red flannel in linseed oil and bind on to the back and chest. Repeat whenever the child coughs (*see also* Crowing, *below*).

## CROUP

Many of the cures recommended for whooping cough (*below*) apply in cases of croup. Light doses of treatments for coughs in adults are used also (*see* Crowing, *below*; *and* Coughing, *under* Respiratory Disorders).

## CROWING

A frightening *crowing* sound can occur during teething or while the child is suffering from paroxysms associated with croup. Pull the tongue forward to open the windpipe and splash cold water on the face and head. Then give the child a hot bath, adding mustard and salt to the water. Keep splashing cold water on the head. If the breathing is still difficult, shake the child or slap its back and buttocks (*see* Croup, *above*).

## DIPHTHERIA

Isolate the patient. Lay flat on the back in a bed with no pillow. Some remedies in Throat, Fever, and Headaches and Migraine (*under* Head) may help.

## ECZEMA

- Mix cabbage juice with unsalted butter and apply.
- Apply fresh cream, buttermilk or curds mixed with honey.
- Avoid using soap for washing the child.
- Drink goat's milk

### FLATULENCE

- Boil caraway seeds or a pinch of ginger in the child's food.

### HERNIA

- Select an ash plant that has never been touched by a slash-hook or any other cutting instrument. Split it and hold it apart with wedges until it is the width of the child. Pass the child through it, remove the wedges and bind it back into its original state. As the sapling grafts together, the hernia will disappear.

### INDIGESTION

- Take a fistful each of hawthorn leaves and purple clover blossom. Boil and strain. Allow to cool, then drink the liquid. Rub the strained vegetable matter on the palms of the hand and the soles of feet.

### MEASLES

If feverish, a child suffering from measles should be kept warm in bed in a darkened room and sponged with warm water occasionally. Kneeling in front of a crucifix before dawn, the parent should say the following prayer three times for three mornings:

'The child has the measles,' said
John the Baptist.

'A short time before it is well,'
said God's Son.
'When is that,' asked John.
'Sunday morning, before dawn,'
said God's Son.

The measles will disappear before the next Sunday.
**Others treatments:**

- Pulverise a garlic clove and mix into pig's lard.
  Place the mixture in a stone jar over a low heat
  where it will sweat. Leave overnight and use as
  an ointment.
- Boil nettles and drink the liquid.
- Make a paste of sheep's dung and fresh milk.
  Rub all over the body.
- Sting the body with nettles.

## MENINGITIS

Keep the child in a darkened room. Give castor oil
as a purgative once only; then feed with nothing
but milk and beef tea. Place a cold stone or a pig's
bladder full of cold water on the head. Use a blister
pack on the neck.

## RICKETS

- Feed the child with whey and blood from raw
  meat.
- Pulverise raw rhubarb and mix with limewater
  and water from a 'brown' stream (i.e. with iron
  content in its waters). Give to drink.

RINGWORM

- Apply the blood of a Keogh.
- Apply a white soda-bread poultice until cured.
- Make a poultice of elder pith and fresh cream. Apply each day for a week.
- Make the Sign of the Cross on the affected area with straw from the Christmas crib.
- Strap a horse's saddle on the patient.
- Dab on friar's balsam each day for a week.
- Mix bread-soda into turpentine and apply.
- Mix goose excrement with rendered hog's fat and apply.
- Dip a finger in ink or linseed oil. First, rub the finger around the circumference of the affected area. Then make the Sign of the Cross along its diameter.
- Apply a mixture of lard and pipe dottle or ash.

SEASICKNESS

Before baptism, parents placed three drops of sea water on a baby's tongue, which would give it lifelong immunity from seasickness.

SKIN INFLAMMATION (IMPETIGO)

If there are crusts on the scalp, shave off the hair. Clean the crusts and apply a mixture of cow's urine and dung or a poultice of oatmeal and buttermilk.

**Other treatments:**

- Render suet. When cool, mix in mercury and apply.

## WHOOPING COUGH

To cure whooping cough, parents put a donkey's
halter on the child and then led it three times
around a pigsty. They then prayed. Sometimes one
parent stood at the door of the sty and called on
the pigs to take the malady, saying '*Seo dhíbh an
triuch*' ('Here is the whooping cough'). The
procedure was also recommended for mumps.
*See* Throat.

County Cavan parents brought their children to
drink water from a skull believed to have been that
of a bishop. The skull was located for periods in
houses along the border with County Meath before
it disappeared. Allegedly, it was taken to England. If
a couple of the same surname married and if a child
ate the final morsel from each one's breakfast, its
whooping cough would disappear. Any man riding a
white horse could tell a distraught parent what to
give the patient.

Feeding the patient the leftovers from a ferret's
meal, sheep's droppings boiled in milk or donkey's
milk were some of the more repulsive cures.

**Other treatments:**

- Cook a mouse and pulverise. Add to some
  food the child likes and feed to the child.
- Follow the advice given by the rider of a
  piebald horse.
- Feed the child bread baked or butter churned
  by a married couple named Mary and Joseph.

- Boil sundew or camomile in donkey's milk and give to the child to drink.
- Pass the child under the foal of an ass three times.
- Hang a 'hairy molly' (caterpillar maturing into a butterfly) around the patient's neck.

## WORMS

Before regular dosing with castor oil, 'worm powders' and Californian 'Syrup of Figs' came to torment the children of careful parents, they drank a half pint of limewater or boiled nettle juice each day for a week.

*Et verbum carum factum est* (and the word was made flesh) is a line from the Angelus. County Leitrim parents kept a 'gospel' containing the line as a cure. With this talisman they made the Sign of the Cross over a glass of water and had the child drink the water.

Healers had a secret prayer, which they said while applying butter or lard to the throat.

**Others treatments:**
- Eat oatmeal bread.
- Smell roasting meat while it is cooking.
- Chew tobacco and swallow its juice.
- Pulverise and boil fern root. Drink when cool.
- Tie a knotted cord around the stomach (*sníomh na péiste,* worm or reptile's twist).

SEVEN

# CONCEPTION, CHILDBIRTH AND FEMALE COMPLAINTS

In 1305, Bernard de Gordon (*c.* 1260–1318), a French physician, wrote *Lilium Medicinae*. Some anonymous Irish doctor translated it into Irish in 1450. A few folk healers, particularly in the period between the fifteenth and the eighteenth centuries, went to the trouble of studying this work and other old medical documents. Thereafter, they had no inhibitions about advising on sexual problems. They disapproved of immoderate sexual intercourse, suggesting that it caused weakness, infirmity and premature ageing. Moderate intercourse, on the other hand, brought happiness and joy to the soul, increased the appetite, dissipated anxiety, quelled anger and induced pleasant sleep.

## BREASTS

Massaging with butter could cure a sore breast if accompanied by the prayer:

'Son of God, see the swelling in this woman's breast. Mary who bore Him,

see it. Mary and King of Heaven
let this woman be healed.'

CONCEPTION

'She's as bitter as a barren woman' was a cruel Irish
saying, because people frowned on a couple who
were without offspring after a number of years of
marriage. One of the reasons for the brouhaha that
occurred when Brinsley MacNamara (1890–1963)
wrote *The Valley of the Squinting Windows* was his
controversial reference to the barren wife of a
butcher in Garradrimna, the author's fictitious
village that people of Delvin, County Westmeath,
took to be theirs:

> She was the hardest woman in
> Garradrimna. Her childlessness had made
> her so. She was beginning to grow stale
> and withered, and anything in the nature
> of love or marriage, with their possible
> results, was to her a constant source of
> affliction and annoyance.

Some women blamed the fairies for their
barrenness. A few wondered if they had mistakenly
eaten barrenwort, a herb thought to cause sterility.
Others wondered if their condition was a
punishment from God, and suffered much mental
anguish as a result. Men never seemed to be held
responsible and so the unfortunate women went on

pilgrimages to pray that God would allow them to give birth. They walked barefoot around the rough penitential beds of Lough Derg (Saint Patrick's Purgatory), County Donegal, or climbed The Reek (Croagh Patrick, near Louisburg, County Mayo). Sneering male neighbours guessed why they went on the pilgrimage and made bawdy comments over their glasses in shebeens. More sympathetic souls held their tongues – they would have liked to offer condolences but did not dare. Some suggestions to aid conception were comic.

**Treatments:**

- Place the bed in a north–south direction or running in line with the floorboards.
- Have intercourse when the tide is on the way in.
- Sew seed from a dock into a sachet and tie it to the right arm of the barren woman.
- The woman should sprinkle sugar on the testicles of a fox and roast them in a pot-oven. She should eat them before the main meal each day for three days.
- Have intercourse when there is a full moon or during its last quarter.
- Visit Saint Brigid's Well, Brideswell, County Roscommon, where a barren daughter of Red Hugh O'Neill was made fertile.
- Sleep on Saint Patrick's Bed, Croagh Patrick.
- Drink waters from a spa near Wexford town (*see* Jaundice, *under* Blood Disorders).

- Husband and wife should pray at the twin wells named after Saint Enda on Inishmore, the largest of the Aran Islands in Galway Bay.

CONTRACEPTION

Despite the restrictions of the Catholic Church, Irish folk cures included methods of contraception, which may be one reason why healers were out of favour with the Church authorities.

The woman was advised to catch a male weasel and castrate it while it was still alive. She then got a small piece of skin from a gander and stitched the weasel's testicles into it. She ran a string through this and kept it hanging about her neck at all times – particularly during intercourse. (Weasel words replacing pillow talk, perhaps!)

Another practice concerned newlyweds. On their wedding day, if anyone did not want them to have offspring, they knotted a kerchief and kept it knotted overnight.

**Other methods:**

- Have intercourse only when the tide is ebbing.
- Have intercourse only during the first quarter of the moon.
- The male should infuse a small amount of the herb barrenwort and drink it. He should take care not to take too much because that could cause sterility (*see* Conception, *above*).

DELIVERY

There was a cavity in a large stone of Saint Loman's Church on Inishmore in Lough Gill, County Sligo. By standing in it and turning around three times, a pregnant woman would have a safe delivery. Lying on Saint Kevin's Bed, a stone in Glendalough, County Wicklow, or placing her head in Saint Olan's Cap, near Coachford, County Cork (*see also* Period Pains, *below*; *and* Head) offered a similar assurance. Drinking water collected in Saint Columcille's Pillow on Tory Island, off the Donegal coast, or chewing clay scraped from his birthplace in Gartan, also County Donegal, assured a safe delivery.

*Teampall na bFir* (Men's Church) stood on Inishmurray Island, off the Sligo coast. A pillarstone there contained a number of holes. In a difficult ritual, a pregnant woman knelt before the stone and, placing thumbs and fingers in these holes, she pulled herself up. This would prevent her dying in childbirth. A fungus formed on growing rye (*claviceps purpurea*) contained ergot and was used by a midwife to contract the womb and to prevent bleeding after delivery.

IMPOTENCE

- Prepare a quarter ounce each of snakeroot, saffron and salt of wormwood. Mix with two ounces of cochineal, one of gentian root and the rind of ten oranges. Steep all in a quart of brandy for at least a day. Use when required.

## LACTATION

Pilgrims to the Holy Land brought home a chalky substance scraped from the wall of the Milk Grotto near Bethlehem where, tradition tells, Mary's milk spilled during lactation. Swallowing the powder increased a mother's milk yield.

**Other treatments:**

- Swallow the juice of milkwort.
- Dry the placenta. Pulverise and eat some of it.
- Rub part of the placenta on the breasts.

## MENOPAUSE

Hot flushes associated with the menopause called for a complicated remedy. Pulverise saffron, lign-aloes and rose stems. Place in rose-water and mix. Soak a linen garment in it and, when dry, wear it.

## MENSTRUATION

The Bible is hard on women. According to Leviticus 15: 9–31, in contemporary English versions:

> When a woman has her monthly period, she remains unclean for seven days, and if you touch her, you must take a bath, but you remain unclean until evening. Anything

that she rests on or sits on is also unclean, and if you touch either of these, you must wash your clothes and take a bath, but you still remain unclean until evening. Any man who has intercourse with her during this time becomes unclean for seven days, and anything he rests on is also unclean.

Any woman who has a flow of blood outside her regular monthly period is unclean until it stops, just as she is during her monthly period. Anything that she rests on or sits on during this time is also unclean, just as it would be during her period. If you touch either of these, you must wash your clothes and take a bath, but you still remain unclean until evening.

Seven days after the woman gets well, she will be considered clean. On the eighth day, she must bring either two doves or two pigeons to the front of my sacred tent and give them to a priest. He will offer one of the birds as a sacrifice for sin and the other as a sacrifice to please me; then I will consider the woman completely clean.

When one of you is unclean, you must stay away from the rest of the community of Israel. Otherwise, my sacred tent will become unclean, and the whole nation will die.

The influence of this biblical text has been apparent down through the centuries. Menstruation was not discussed in Irish homes but there was a tacit understanding in ancient times that a menstruating woman could destroy crops and taint food. She avoided becoming involved in separating milk, or churning, because if she did, the milk would sour and the butter would be dangerous to eat. She did not handle or prepare food.

Some mothers gave quite alarming advice to their daughters, warning them never to walk in long grass, for example, because their condition would attract lizards to run up the legs and attack. They should also avoid placing their feet in cold water because this could send the blood to the head and cause madness.

Wise women and men offered an even more frightening warning – that having intercourse during menstruation led to the next conception bringing forth a monster, perhaps an infant covered with hair or having extra limbs. Perhaps a whimsical Irish twist on this nonsense was that the next child would be a redhead.

A folk remedy for excessive menstruation recommended taking five grains of powdered ergot of rye every four hours. It was also believed that a spa near Wexford town (*see* Jaundice, *under* Blood Disorders) cured excessive menstruation.

## PERIOD PAINS

There were many remedies for period pains. For example, women were advised to avoid washing hair, and avoid swimming. And a visit to Saint Olan's Cap near Coachford, County Cork, was said to cure them (*see* Head).

## PLACENTA

The wise woman or midwife often burned the placenta and listened. She could tell from the number of spits during the burning how many more children her patient would have. If it burned for a long time, the newborn child would have a long life.

Some fathers buried the placenta under an elder bush. (*See also* Lactation, *above*.)

## PREGNANCY AND LABOUR

The expectant mother should keep a scrap of skin from the stomach of a corpse in her clothing to ensure a healthy pregnancy. To ensure an easy labour, she should eat fish brains frequently.

**Other treatments for labour:**

- The husband carries a heavy slab of stone over his head around the kitchen. His wife should be able to see him when he passes her bedroom door. This eases her pain.

- If the hair of the woman in labour is long, the midwife should twist it into a ball and stuff it into her mouth. The struggle to breathe helps the delivery. A ball of wool will have the same effect.

## SEX OF CHILD

To conceive a girl, the woman was advised to turn slowly on to her right side after intercourse. If she wanted a boy, she turned on her left side. To confirm this during pregnancy, she baked a cake using her own milk instead of buttermilk. A hard crust suggested a boy and a soft one, a girl. (*See also* my *Irish Customs* in this Gill & Macmillan series.)

If a parent brought its newborn infant to Saint Brendan's Well at Kilmeena, County Mayo, and dipped it in the water, its sex would change. A story tells that the O'Malley sept would be extinct but for the well's power. All its male adults and children were killed in an attempt to eliminate the sept but, later, one girl was dipped in the well and became a male as she reached adolescence.

EIGHT

# FEVER

Irish people referred to fever as 'night fire' or *éagruas* (infirmity). A son born after his father's death could cure fever by saying a particular prayer but many households without such a son used it also.

> Earth fire is hot; hell's fire is hotter, but
> the love of Mary is above all. Who will
> quench this fire? Who will heal the sick?
> Let the Fire of God destroy the Evil One.

A patient suffering from fever would be helped to a sitting position in bed. A member of his family would raise his arms in the form of a cross, sprinkle holy water on his head and pray to Saint Michael.

If that did not work, they got a healer to 'peg [throw] the stones'. He placed a spell on three stones. Throwing one away, he said, 'This is the head of the fever.' Then he cast another, and said, 'This is the heart of the fever.' While casting the third, he said, 'This is the back of the fever.' Then he prayed, 'In the name of the Blessed Trinity, give the man peace.' Next, the healer breathed on a spoonful of butter and got the patient to rub it on as many parts of his body as he could reach. Then he asked the patient to hold a sprig of yarrow in his right hand while he slept. The patient did not know that this would signify his fate. If it withered overnight, he would die.

Unscrupulous carers gave the patient a drink (preferably elderberry wine) but kept some in the glass or cup. They would offer this to someone else (perhaps an enemy), and so 'pass on' the fever.

If fever was present in a County Kerry community, every family that was spared underwent a pilgrimage. They walked from Wether's Well near Tralee to Saint Brigid's Well at Ballyheige. Usually, they also visited Saint Macadaw's Church and Well at the foot of Trisk Mountain near Glenderry.

**Other treatments:**

- Allow an incoming tide to wash over the feet of the patient. When the tide ebbs, it will take the fever with it.
- Place the patient on a sandy shore.
- Eat small fish found in the stomachs of larger fish.
- Boil spikes of spore-cases from club moss. Drink the liquid and place the remainder on the brow.
- Drink copious amounts of water.
- Drink moderate amounts of alcoholic beverages.
- Drink the juice of cow dung.

- Pulverise dandelion stems. Pour boiling water over them. Sip a small amount at a time.

## AGUE

Ague is an old name for malarial or other fever. In Ireland people believed it developed from regular walking on marshy land or bogs. Ocean-going seamen kept lance-leaved Peruvian bark on board. They treated ague by pulverising one ounce and boiling it in one pint of water. After straining and cooling, the patient drank two tablespoonfuls when he got a bout of shivering.

**Other treatments:**

- Rub the back with equal parts of turpentine and rum. Ensure regular bowel movement.
- Eat a live spider.
- Drink water from Tobar Halamóg, Salterstown, County Louth.

NINE

# HEAD

## HEADACHES AND MIGRAINE

Sufferers from headaches and migraine have always visited certain holy wells and stones associated with inexplicable successes in curing. Such places usually have some connection with a saint who lived in the area or who passed through it.

People still visit Saint Hugh's Headache Stone in Rahugh, County Westmeath, and pray at his holy well. Tradition tells that a hollow in the stone came about when the saint carried it on his head from his home place at Killare beside the Hill of Uisneach. Some attest to being cured of severe migraine by placing the head against the hollow in the stone and praying at the saint's well nearby. My own wife is among them.

Similar practices are associated with Saint Olan's Cap (*Caipín*), which crowns an ogham pillarstone in Aghabullogue, near Coachford, County Cork. It cures headaches and period pains. A priest once removed the stone because of its phallic shape but locals replaced it. Another stone nearby is said to bear the imprint of the saint's feet.

People tell of the imprint of Saint Patrick's head and feet appearing on two stone slabs near Oranmore, County Galway. Kneeling and placing feet and head in the relevant hollows was said to bring relief. Bathing the head in water from a hollow in Saint Ciaran's Stone at Clonmacnoise, County Offaly, was also beneficial.

Sitting in Saint Fechin's Bath in Fore, County Westmeath, or drinking 'the water that won't boil' from his well also brought cures. A story tells how a disbeliever tried to boil the water, failed to get even a puff of steam and suffered from headaches for the rest of his life.

The grave of Saint Barry is said to be in Kilbarry, County Roscommon. People suffering from headache took clay from it and rubbed it on their heads (*see also* introduction to Stomach).

Other wells associated with headache cures include Saint Colman's, Kilcolman, County Waterford; Saint Brigid's, Kilranelagh, County Carlow, and Saint Ciaran's, Castlekeeran, County Meath.

On Saint Brigid's Day, 1 February, people tied Saint Brigid's ribbon (*Ribín Bhríde*) to doorknobs; then they kept it to wind around the head to cure headaches (or around the throat for a sore throat or tonsilitis). Snuff left over after a wake could cure headaches also. And people exercised care when they disposed of hair clippings, because if a bird used them in nest-building, the owner would suffer from headaches until the next nesting season.

Some healers recited a Latin invocation to the Holy Lord God of Sabbath before rubbing spittle on the temples and head of patients while saying the Our Father three times. They concluded by making the Sign of the Cross and outlining the letter 'U' on the head with the spittle. This may have suggested the Latin '*Ultimo*' ([in the] last).

*See also*, Holy Wells.

**Other treatments:**

- Leave brown paper to steep in vinegar, a mustard paste, Burgundy wine, *poitín* or whiskey. Place on the head, preferably after shaving off the hair.
- Collect hoar frost on the morning of Saint Brigid's Day (1 February) and rub it on the forehead.
- Boil lavender blooms in water and drink.
- Bind the head with a strip of a sheet that has been used as a shroud.

## ADENOIDS

Lay the patient down and drip salted water into each nostril. He should then inhale deeply through the nose and exhale through the mouth.

## APOPLEXY

Lay patient down. Turn on side and place a wet towel on the head.

## BALDNESS

Advice on applying some of the treatments prescribed for baldness ended with a warning to

wear gloves to prevent hair growing on the hands.
There's confidence!

**Treatments:**

- Place a live eel in a bottle. Cork it and bury the bottle in a dunghill until the contents become an oily liquid. Rub this into the scalp daily.

- To within an inch from its brim, fill a small earthenware pot with mice. Pack clay on to the remaining space and leave in the ashpit under the hearth for a year. Apply to the scalp.

- Put six mice in a sealed earthenware container and place at the back of the hearth; then build the fire in front of the container. Open it after six days and massage the scalp with the contents.

- Rub the scalp with a sliced onion.

- Rub on clay from Teach Dorcha, Kilbarry, County Roscommon (*see* introduction to Stomach and Bowels).

- Burn a raven and boil the ashes with mutton fat. Rub on the scalp when cool.

- Pass urine into a goat's bladder. Hang in the chimney-stack until the urine evaporates and the bladder is brittle; then pulverise. Halve an onion, sprinkle with the powder, and rub into the scalp.

- Boil some mice and worms. Mix to a paste and apply.

- Burn sally rods. Mix the ash with turpentine

and a boar's fat until it has a thick, pasty texture. Apply nightly.

- Blister the scalp by applying a hot poultice.
- Rub in bone marrow from a cow.
- Cut a raw onion in two and rub the scalp with the inner surface.

## CATARRH

In a pint of rainwater, dissolve two ounces each of bread soda, salt and pulverised borax. Using one part of the solution to two of water, sniff up the nose regularly. Double the dose at bedtime.

## DANDRUFF

Wash head in warm water. Rub in sulphur ointment. Soak any crusts with linseed or almond oil. Repeat daily until dandruff disappears.

## DIZZINESS

- Boil lavender blooms in water and drink regularly.

## EARACHE

*See* Organs.

## HANGOVER

Dubliners cured their hangovers by drinking from a spa well beside the Weavers' Hall in the Coombe. The trouble was, they often visited a nearby tavern afterwards.

**Other treatments:**

- Have a 'hair of the dog that bit you', i.e. take a 'cure', or one more alcoholic drink.
- Boil lavender blooms in water and drink.

HEAD LICE

*See* Skin.

TEN

# HERBS

In Irish mythology, Dian Cécht was a celebrated physician to King Nuada. Dian Cécht's son Miach became more proficient in medicine and was murdered by his jealous father. Miach's sister, Airme, visited her brother's grave and found 365 herbs growing on it. She reckoned that each one represented one day of the year, but on investigation discovered that each herb's root was growing in a different muscle, bone, sinew or organ of Miach's body. She gathered them up and made notes on their origins. King Nuada found the papers, neatly categorised; he tossed them in the air and the winds spread them around the woods, fields and glens of Ireland. Many must have been lost, because later, just seven plants formed the basis of folk cures. They were elder bark, eyebright, foxglove, groundsel, hawthorn buds, ivy, and the herb that was also an amulet, vervain.

In basic folk medicine the herbalist – usually a woman (*bean na luibheanna*, herb woman) – mixed and pounded these plants before rolling them into nine balls. The patient ate the balls and washed them down with water taken from a bog hole and boiled in a pot containing a coin and an elf-stone. Only the wise woman knew how to administer certain herbs and it was dangerous for others to attempt using them. For example, hemlock, though poisonous, was used with care in poultices and ointments, or as a plaster. She used vague names for certain herbs and only she understood them and their qualities. She had to be skilled, because the Devil had a habit of fashioning fake plants to look exactly like the authentic ones. *Luibh Mór* (big herb), for instance, healed and also acted as an amulet. It could cure the dreadful, delirious urge to keep travelling, which gripped a person after stepping on fairy grass, the 'stray sod', or *fód seachrán* (lit. 'wandering sod').

The name of the Blessed Virgin Mary appeared among the names of herbs: *lus na Maighdine Muire, aiteann Mhuire, coineall Mhuire, crobhán Mhuire, dréimire Mhuire* and *seamair Mhuire* – the blessed herb. Respectively, these translate as the plant of the Virgin Mary, and Mary's furze, Mary's candle, Mary's small hand, Mary's ladder and Mary's (four-leafed) clover. Herbs or plants had local names too: fairy potatoes, fairy fingers, fairy flax, robin-run-the-hedge and piss-a-beds.

The herb woman also knew of certain herbs that lost their power if plucked by hand. She solved this difficulty ingeniously by tying the required plant to an animal's foot and urging the beast forward until it was uprooted. Many a wise woman collected some herbs by the light of a candle held by a dead man's hand. She did her work at midnight when the moon was full.

Some activities struck fear into country folk. In west Galway long ago it was common practice to see a close relative of a patient plucking some anonymous herb at dawn and uttering a prescribed incantation while holding it up to the newly risen sun. If nothing happened, the patient would recover but if it withered, he or she would die.

Besides the seven prominent herbs, other flora provided ingredients for folk cures. Mosses or mould from stones, particularly when they were found in church ruins or beside holy wells, featured regularly. Yarrow was widely used to cure certain ailments, and was also used as a preventative when sewn into the hem of a garment.

On Saint John's Eve (23 June, Midsummer Eve) country people collected Saint John's wort, yarrow, figwort and foxglove for medicinal use during the following year. They also stored bark, pith, leaves, fruit and buds from trees, especially the elder, oak, elm, blackthorn, willow and ash. Gathering this material was not confined to Saint John's Eve, but the herbs were considered more potent if collected then. Care was exercised with Saint John's wort because an overdose could be poisonous. It had many uses, whether drunk or used as a poultice or lotion. In the year 2002 the Irish government banned across-the-counter sale of preparations containing the herb. It had become known as 'nature's Prozac' because clinical trials had shown it to be as potent as some antidepressants.

Herbs collected on May Day could heal or harm, depending on whether the gatherer invoked Satan or the Blessed Trinity. The seven herbs that could kill were eyebright, mallow, Saint John's wort, self-help, speedwell, vervain and yarrow. Originally, the fairies explained their uses to mortals for malefic purposes. When they were on the point of death, holders of the secrets could pass them on to the eldest of a family. Persons carrying a potion of this sort could never look back or pass on the container to anyone except the person for whom it was intended.

Writers and physicians have written books and theses about herbs and herb remedies but the bulk of knowledge available on their use in Irish folk cures was handed down orally. Much of it has been lost forever and very few places still exist where a local healer, a parent or a sufferer would prepare a remedy from herbs or plants gathered in the countryside.

ELEVEN

# HOLY WELLS

Unkind critics of a gaudily dressed woman would often say 'She's like a bush at a holy well', because, to vouch for a cure, grateful people left strips of clothing, crutches, rosary beads, pieces of bandage and assorted rags on and around bushes and trees close by a healing well. From earliest times, water has symbolised life. Seeking supernatural assistance in illness by drinking water is a tradition that dates back to the arrival of Christianity and, in some cases, to the pre-Christian period.

A pattern (*patrún*, patron) often celebrated a pilgrimage to a holy well. As the name implies, it was a day to honour the local patron saint; a day when Roman Catholic clergy celebrated Mass in a nearby church or at the saint's shrine. Many pattern days coincided with the festivals of *Lughnasa, Domhnach Chrom Dhubh* or Garland Sunday. Despite the celebratory nature of all these patterns, the underlying idea of the pilgrimage was to obtain a cure for oneself, a relative or friend. Outside of pattern days, of course, people still paid private visits, and many a sorrowful soul prayed quietly for a cure. (For more on patterns, see my *Irish Customs* in this Gill & Macmillan series.)

During his visit, the pilgrim walked around the well in a sunwise direction, reciting prayers at stone 'stations'. 'Paying Rounds' was an accepted ritual. Afterwards, he drank the waters or washed affected parts of his body with it. Then he took a stone from the well and scraped a cross on it with another sharp-edged stone.

Lady Day (25 March, the feast of the Annunciation) attracted large crowds to Our Lady's Well at Killargue, between Drumkeerran and Drumshanbo, County Leitrim, and to Lady's Well in Athenry, County Galway. On Easter Monday, County Clare pilgrims went to Scattery Island in the Shannon estuary, near Kilrush, where Saint Senan founded a monastery. They knelt on the stony shoreline and prayed but made up for their hardship later with lavish refreshments and exuberant entertainment.

Dublin had its pattern of Saint John's Well, Kilmainham. Being a city event, it was quite elaborate. Pedlars erected stalls and sold patchwork quilts, sheep fleeces and assorted drapery. Caterers lit fires and boiled mutton, crubeens and vegetables. The event became problematic due to excessive drinking and fighting, which, in 1710, forced the Irish House of Commons to declare it a menace and threaten whippings, fines and even incarceration for misbehaviour. In Dublin county, Saint Maelruan's pattern on 7 July was held in Tallaght. The saint's name was corrupted to 'Moll Rooney's', and roisterers, carrying an effigy of

'Moll' went from house to house, collecting money and taking occupants onto the street to dance.

Irishtown, or 'The Butts', in Kilkenny held a similar pattern but the city's portreeve ordered an end to the custom in 1608. A major pattern took place at Saint James's Well, Callan, County Kilkenny, on 26 July.

Water taken from holy wells on Easter Sunday had special curative powers. Those with a history of successful cures were called Sunday's Wells (*Tobar Rí an Domhnaigh*, Well of the King of Sunday). Observing a rising sun while standing beside one was beneficial to health and good fortune, particularly on Easter Sunday morning.

Tradition declared that from midnight on Saint John's Eve (23 June) until 1 a.m. on Saint John's Day water in all wells named after Saint John (the Baptist) boiled. If collected before 2 a.m. it would cure any ailment.

There were legends attached to most holy wells. For example, Saint Finian of Waterville was said to have suffered from leprosy when he visited Killemlagh in County Kerry. He took a fern from the ruins of a church there and, after stroking his sores with it, he was cured. Sufferers from king's evil (scrofula, tubercular glands in the neck) visit the site. The name 'king's evil' also comes from folklore. Saint Edward the Confessor was King of England from 1042 to 1066. His touch cured sufferers from scrofula and usually he hung a gold medal around their necks. The custom ended with the death of Queen Anne in 1714. By then the practice had spread to France, where it continued until 1775. Louis XVI is credited with touching 2,400 sufferers on his coronation day alone. Cynics claim that the gold medal attracted more than genuine cases!

A protester washed his dog's leg in a popular well at Kilteevan, County Roscommon, and the water disappeared. Any holy well would dry up if desecrated but its curative powers would then be transferred to a nearby tree. People could stick pins or hammer coins into the tree where previously they drank the well water. This practice destroyed the 'Tree that won't Burn', one of the 'Seven Wonders of Fore' in County Westmeath. Fore had pilgrimages and patterns on Saint Peter's Day (29 June), Saint John's Day and on Saint Fechin's Day (20 January).

'Eye wells' cured sight loss or eye infections. Some cured sight deficiencies in animals — but at the risk of the owner becoming infected. Examples include a well on the County Cavan slope of Slieve Anierin (*Sliabh an Iarainn*, Hill of Iron) and wells called *Tobar na Súl* (Eye Well) near Ballymena, County Antrim, on *Sliabh Sneacht[a]* (Snow Mountain), County Donegal, and at Glendahalin, Ballyheigue, County Kerry. Saint Brigid's Well, near Ardagh, County Longford, was another eye well but it also cured 'delicate' people, a euphemism often used for tuberculosis sufferers. If it dried up, people used moss from its stones to treat whooping cough.

Saint Brigid is associated with eye wells because of two legends. One tells how, after a persistent suitor admired their beauty, she plucked out her eyes and threw them at him. This halted his advances and she had her eyes restored later by bathing them in a well at Killinagh, near Blacklion, County Cavan. (The story may also provide a clue to the origin of Killinagh's cursing stones.) Brigid also befriended a blind nun in her Kildare monastery. She miraculously gave her colleague sight, but when the nun saw the beauty of the countryside, she asked to be returned to her blind state. She reasoned that the beauty around her might distract her from prayer.

Saint Craven's Eye Well near Ennistymon, County Clare, was famous throughout Munster and Connaught.

On 25 March, the feast of the Annunciation (Lady Day), pilgrims visited Tobar Muire (Mary's Well) near Dundalk, County Louth. On their knees, they shuffled westward around the well before drinking from it. This, they believed, could cure ailments and forgive sin.

Not strictly a well, but water collected on a tomb near a church ruin at Newtown Bridge,

County Meath, cured warts when combined with the pin-pointing method (*see* Warts, *under* Skin). Other holy wells that cured warts included: Mulhuddart, County Dublin, and Holywood, County Wicklow.

Saint Finian's Trough, possibly a monastery lavabo, in Clonard, County Meath, always holds water. Its curative powers include ridding patients of warts. Water held in the hollow of a 'wart stone' in Beaghmore, Carrigallen, County Leitrim, possessed the same curative properties.

Saint Patrick's Well near Rathvilly, County Carlow, had a large flat stone above it. It bore an imprint roughly resembling a foot. From it, tradition states, the saint stepped into Knockpatrick, County Kildare, five miles distant. Water from the hollow had curative properties. (A field nearby has a 'Bow' stone, i.e. a stone on which the Banshee sat.)

Saint Colman's Well on the slopes of the Hill of Allen in County Kildare attracted pilgrims up to the mid-nineteenth century and Saint Brigid's Well at Tully, near Kildare town, still does. Trinity Well at Carbury, the source of the River Boyne, is another holy well. Cures have been claimed from all three.

Drinking water from certain holy wells cured toothache. County Dublin had Saint Senan's Well at Slade, Saint Mobhi's at Grange and Saint Catherine's at Drumcondra. County Kilkenny had Saint Fiachre's, near Graiguenamanagh (Ullard) and County Leitrim had Saint Brigid's near Ballinamore, where doing a round of the stations in the cemetery nearby could have the same result.

Another well named after Saint Brigid in Graigenaspidogue, County Carlow, cured a number of ailments, and in the same county, Saint Brigid's Well at Kilranelagh cured headaches.

If sprinkled around a garden, water from Saint Senan's Well in Kiltenane, County Clare, rid soil of wireworm. Another Clare well, Saint Michael's at Querrin, cured a cripple on one occasion. People came across the sea from the Aran Islands to Saint Brigid's Well at Moher, County Clare on 1 August each year. The elaborate Saint Brigid's Well or Tub (Dabhach *or* Daigh Bhríde) is still surrounded by paraphernalia of cured patients. Six outer and inner 'rounds' demanded six recitals of the Lord's Prayer and six Hail Marys each. The exercise ended with the kissing of a cross and drinking from the well.

Seafaring people kept a supply of water from Saint Ciaran's Well on Clare Island in their homes. Drinking some before going to sea prevented seasickness.

Killare and Tullaghan in County Westmeath have wells dedicated to Saint Brigid. Parents bring children with whooping cough to drink water from Tobar Bríd (Brigid's Well) in Darragh, County Limerick. They also bring home moss from the stones of the well, boil it in milk and coax the child to drink it. County Dublin wells, Saint Mo-Chuda's (or Cárthách) at Bunnow, Gregan's at Garristown and Chincough (or Chink) at Portrane also cured whooping cough.

A number of cures have been attributed to drinking from Saint Laserian's Well at Old Leighlin, near Leighlinbridge, County Carlow. Ballygorey Well close to Tullow was associated with cures for rheumatism.

There was a 'curtsy stone' at Cullen Well in Cork where pilgrims bent their knees during the prescribed stations. Saint Latiaran is said to have planted a hawthorn bush there and it became a popular site for post-pattern faction fights between the Daithini and the Gearaltaigh.

Saint Finbar had an island hermitage in Lough Gougane Barra, near Inchigeela, County Cork. Surrounded by high mountains, the isolated spot was ideal for his prayer and penance. A fierce serpent lived there until Finbar banished it to a small lake on the top of Mount Gabriel, near Skull. On his feast day, 25 September, a major Munster pattern was held and pilgrims came from far and near to pray and drink Gougane Barra's water, believing it had curative powers.

Saint Killian (c. 640–89) of Mullagh in County Cavan became famous in Würzburg, Germany. At Mullagh and in their home country, Germans celebrate an annual 'Kilianfest'. His holy well at Cloughballybeg was the location of one of the oldest patterns in Ireland. It took place on his feast day, 8 July. Pilgrims have claimed cures for a number of ailments.

Saint Michael's Well, Ballinskelligs, County Kerry, cured the crippled, blind and deaf. Tobar na nGealt (Well of Lunatics) near Kilgobban, County Kerry, cured mental illness.

Saint Bernard's Wells at Rathkeale and at Ardpatrick and the Blessed Well of Ballingarry are all in County Limerick. They cured warts and other maladies.

Father Moore's Well on the Curragh's edge at Rathbride is more modern. It is said that this priest performed miracles, and when he died in 1826, visits to a well near his cottage began. Wearing his hat for an instant became an accepted cure for headaches.

Those mentioned above are just a handful of Ireland's holy wells. Some have dried up or have disappeared. In almost every parish in the country there is or has been a holy well and for centuries good people have been visiting them. Many still continue the practice – in hope, in anticipation, often in desperation.

Other holy wells associated with particular ailments receive mention under those headings.

TWELVE

# MENTAL AILMENTS

The Irish had a beautiful and sensitive name for a mentally disadvantaged person. He or she was a *duine le Dia* (person with God) and kind people searched for folk cures for their afflicted relatives. These included crossing a river a number of times, chewing watercress from a holy well or holding a burning turf sod near the mouth and inhaling the smoke. Chronic cases visited Teach Dorcha (Dark House) in Kilbarry, County Roscommon (*see* Stomach). There, the patient slept on straw during the nights of Thursday, Friday and Saturday. On Sunday he attended Mass in the local church.

People brought patients long distances in search of a cure. Perhaps to sit on the Madman's Chair (also Cathaoir Ana, Ana's Chair), a stone on the shore at Dunany Point, near Clogherhead, County Louth. Or to drink water from a stream near Moville, County Donegal.

## AMNESIA
Wealthier people drank white wine laced with pounded frankincense.

## DEPRESSION
If a person became listless, people believed he had 'heart sadness' as a result of receiving a 'fairy blast'.

The healer dealt with this by dousing the patient with 'blast water' while praying: 'In the name of the sword-bearing saint, who has God's strength and who stands by His side, be cured!'

**Other treatments for all forms of depression:**

- Pulverise saffron, lign-aloes and rose stems. Place in rose-water and mix. Soak a linen garment in it and, when dry, wear it.
- Take a trip on the sea, particularly if the water is rough.
- Kill a robin and remove its heart. Stitch it into a sachet, run a cord through it and wear around the neck.

EPILEPSY

Frequent fainting, fits or 'falling sickness' (*an galar póil*) called for burying a tress of the patient's hair and his nail clippings while saying a prayer:

By the power of Mary and the soul of Paul, let the great illness lie in the clay forever.

A similar prayer accompanied a ritual of planting a wooden peg in the ground and winding a cord around it. Both treatments benefited from being performed beside a holy well.

Some healers boiled rue and mixed in nine bone shards from a skeleton's skull. The patient took a teaspoonful every morning while fasting. Like today's course of antibiotics, he had to finish all; otherwise the dead man would come looking for his skull splinters back!

**Other treatments:**

- Boil pulverised garlic in water taken from a mearing stream.
- Wear a gospel containing the opening verse of the Gospel According to Saint John.
- Jump across a stream at dawn, then bathe in it.
- Cut an elder twig into nine pieces, each an inch long. With a needle, run three strands of silk thread through all the pieces, forming a chain. Hang it around the patient's neck, making sure it touches the skin. The charm is only effective as long as it never touches the earth.
- Pass the patient under a donkey nine times.
- Eat cloves of garlic regularly.
- During an attack, loosen clothes around the neck and chest. Place a clean cloth between the teeth to prevent damage to the tongue. Hold in a position so that the patient will not injure himself.

NIGHTMARE

Evil spirits caused nightmares and treatment included wrapping a horseshoe in red flannel and placing it under the pillow.

**Other treatments:**

- Sleep on the back.
- Find a stone with a hole in it. Run a string of wool through the hole and hang over the bed.

THIRTEEN

# MUSCLES, TISSUES AND NERVES

Most people suffering from aches and pains in the back, limbs, tendons, muscles, bones, joints or nerves referred to their 'rheumatism'. Doctors would be more specific. Men working in the fields or in the bog all day would often come home and steep their feet in a basinful of water as hot as they could bear. They would keep the kettle 'on the hob' and reheat the water when it became cooler. They blamed dampness for their complaint. Metal parts of a decayed coffin or its nails were often used to forge rings or bracelets to alleviate muscular pains.

There have been claims that beekeepers never developed rheumatism and so some sufferers allowed bees to sting them. People stung aching limbs with nettles too.

Stones from Tobar na nAingeal (Well of Angels) in County Donegal and water from Lady's Well at Tyrellstown, County Dublin, or from Tobar Finnáin (Finian's Well) on Valentia Island, County Kerry, cured rheumatism, sciatica, aches, pains, sprains and general muscular ailments. Seal oil was regarded as a cure for rheumatism or sprains and there were even rumours that the great Kerry football teams of the past used a concoction containing seal oil for massaging the limbs of their gladiators.

County Wicklow people visited Glendalough to sit in Saint Kevin's Chair. County Westmeath folk preferred to lie in Saint Fechin's Keeve (tub or bath) in Fore, where the saint spent nights in prayer. Saint Cuimin of Conor vouched for this:

> Fechin the generous of Fobhar loved –
> It was no hypocritical devotion –
> To place his meagre rib
> Upon a hard bed without clothes.

Sitting in a sweat house built of stone to ease aches was common in Ulster.

Paddling in seawater or bathing in seaweed relieved muscular aches and pains. Ballybunion, Lisdoonvarna, Bundoran and other holiday resorts had 'spas' and seaweed baths which were also beneficial.

A bog onion has a number of bulbs. One of these soaked in a half pint of water thickened the liquid and provided a useful massaging agent.

The paw of a hare hung around a person's neck on May Day cured ailments of the muscles or joints, such as cramp and rheumatism.

Some people believed that fairy darts caused 'strokes' or stabbing pains. To cure them, they placed some pointed instrument into water, which they then gave to the victim to drink.

A poultice of flax and its tow was a popular painkiller. Sometimes people made them into a paste with a little lard and rubbed it on the affected parts. An old story explained that Jesus once asked for shelter in a house but its owner refused. The man's wife brought the stranger in, however, and allowed Him to eat, drink and rest. The disgruntled owner protested but was suddenly overcome with severe pains. Jesus took some flax and tow, touched the man with them and cured him.

A prayer accompanied the treatment:

In the name of a mild woman and a tough
man and of the Lamb of God, be healed
from your sins and your pains.

DROPSY
- Boil bog broom in a little water and drink the juice.
- Cook a wood-louse or cockroach. Mix into elderberry wine and drink.
- Boil down meadowsweet or nettles from a cemetery. Drink the liquid twice a day.
- Boil nettles gathered in a churchyard and drink the liquid.

GENERAL PAINS
- Massage with unsalted butter or goose grease.
- Apply hot red flannel and keep hot by ironing.

- Pour on copious amounts of cold spring water.
- Apply a poultice of boiled comfrey roots.
- Fry a hedgehog. Rub the grease on the affected area.
- Boil waterlily roots. Thicken with goose grease if necessary to make a paste. Rub the affected part.
- Apply a poultice of damp bog moss or moss from a damp ditch.
- Bathe in Saint Declan's Well, Ardmore, County Waterford.

## GOUT
- Wrap affected joint in red flannel.
- Use any blister pack to cause slight blistering.

## GROWING PAINS
- Apply a poultice of fresh cow dung to aching areas.

## KNEE PAINS
- Tie an eel's skin around the knee.

## LEG CRAMP
- Press the heel of the affected leg hard against the end of the bed or on the floor.
- To cure leg or foot cramps, eat two bananas per day.

## LUMBAGO

- Apply a poultice of crushed nettle leaves.
- Dip red flannel in boiling water. Wring it out. Sprinkle on a few drops of turpentine. Apply to the affected area.

## NEURALGIA

- Apply a plaster of cow dung.
- Heat red flannel and apply.
- Heat black paper and apply.
- Pulverise deadly nightshade (belladonna) and mix two teaspoonfuls of its juices to eight of olive oil. Use as a liniment.
- Pulverise monkshood and add three teaspoonfuls of its juice to two of lard. Use to massage the affected area.

## OEDEMA (FLUID IN TISSUES)

- Boil down meadowsweet or nettles from a cemetery. Chew the solid substance and drink the liquid.

## PULLED MUSCLE

- Tying a weaver's knot or a string of nine knots or a length of red thread around a sprain brought relief. There are still women in the countryside who treat sprains or back pains by winding a strand of brown wool around the calf or ankle and praying:

> The Lord rade and the foal slade.
> He lighted and He righted;
> Set joint to joint and bone to bone,
> And sinew upon sinew.
> In the name of God and the saints,
> Let this person be healed.

The patient must keep wearing the wool until the ailment disappears. I know a woman who claims to have visited eminent surgeons and chiropractors with excruciating back pains. She found no relief until she visited a woman who performed a similar ritual.

A prayer said while holding a pulled muscle went:

> Jesus was travelling over a mountain and
> His horse's foot He sprained. Jesus said,
> 'Blood to blood, bone to bone, nerve to
> nerve and each sinew in its own place.'

The practice of applying wool originated in a legend about Saint Patrick. After being refused permission to ford the Garavogue River at Sligo, he rode around by the shore of Lough Gill. Near Dromahaire, the horse pulled a leg muscle. Patrick manipulated some stones to correct the injury. A custom developed whereby wise women tied pieces of string around one of the stones that became embedded in the ground. Thereafter, they used the string for muscular complaints and backache.

**Other treatments:**

- Mix a half pint of turpentine with two raw eggs. Pour into a two pint, lidded container and shake vigorously until creamy. Add one pint of vinegar, one tablespoonful of ammonia and a camphor ball, if available. Use as an embrocation. The preparation will last for years and is also useful for sore throats.

- Mix three tablespoonfuls of ammonia with two of turpentine and one of camphor spirits. Soak a piece of flannel in the mixture. Secure it on the sprain with a bandage.

- Heat antiphlogistine (take care not to overheat) and smear on brown paper. Apply to sprained area and bandage.

## RHEUMATISM

A healer moves his hands upward over the painful part but never touches it. He utters prescribed phrases in a low voice that the patient should not hear.

Dubliners cured their rheumatism by bathing in a spa well beside the Weavers' Hall in the Coombe.

**Other treatments:**

- Chew boiled seaweed.

- Eat watercress.

- Chew a raw onion.

- Carry a potato, nutmeg or a hazelnut in the pocket.
- Wear a copper bracelet.

## SCIATICA

- Apply a poultice of crushed nettle leaves.
- Wash the affected area in hot water. Mix one ounce of ammonia into a quarter pint of turpentine. Add two ounces of camphorated oil. Shake well and massage the affected area.

## STABBING PAINS

Some people believed that fairy darts caused 'strokes', or stabbing pains. They placed a pointed instrument into water and gave it to the victim to drink.

## STITCH

- Lift and turn a stone in a meadow.
- Rub unsalted butter on the side affected by the stitch, and then make the Sign of the Cross seven times over it.
- Make the Sign of the Cross on the area using a green stone from a stream.
  Rub barley tow (*colg eorna)* on the affected area.

FOURTEEN

# ORGANS

The rituals employed by healers of old were probably most awesome when dealing with internal organs. A patient would know little about these organs or their functions and so the theatricals observed during a visit to the healer impressed all the more.

## BLADDER
*See* Liver, *below; and* Urine.

## BRAIN
Eating fish regularly was thought to be good for the brain.

**Stroke:** Ingest self-heal, a variety of prunella, by any method.

**Water on the brain:** Wrap the head in a lamb's fleece. Cover with oilskin. This will draw off the water.

## CORONARY COMPLAINTS
Romantic heartache was not in Irish people's minds when they referred to '*an crá croí*' (the heart anguish). This was the pain in the chest which is associated nowadays with coronary problems.

A healer first put the patient to bed. He then placed an eggcup, glass or teacup filled with oatmeal on the spot where the pain originated and strapped it in place. On the third, sixth or ninth day (according to local custom) he examined the oatmeal and sometimes gave the patient some oatmeal bread to eat. If the amount of the oatmeal in the vessel diminished, it suggested that a weak heart was using it up and therefore the ailment required more intensive analysis. This involved laying a strip of ribbon about three feet long on a table. Above and below it, the healer laid two threads, each a different colour, then carefully rolled up all three and, invoking the Blessed Trinity, made the Sign of the Cross on chest and back with the roll. Unrolling them then, he studied them. If the threads were in reverse order, the patient would survive.

**Other treatments:**

- A healer utters a secret prayer while pressing a poultice of oatmeal to the heart area.
- Boil foxglove. Sweeten with honey. Allow to cool and drink.
- Chew cloves of garlic.

## EAR COMPLAINTS

**Earache:** With a sharp knife or small cleaver, a healer cut off the horns of a black snail. Even at a distance from the patient, this cured severe earache.

**Other treatments:**

- Apply a wild mustard leaf to the back of the ear.

- Place hot red flannel on the ear and head.
- Heat two drops of laudanum or glycerine on a spoon. Drop into the ear.
- Shear wool from a black sheep and place a small wad in the ear.
- Roast an onion and hold to the ear. Reheat if necessary.
- Drop juice of coltsfoot into the ear.

**Ear Noise (Tinnitus):** A ringing in the ear was a soul in Purgatory calling for assistance. Praying for the soul helped it reach heaven and stopped the 'bell in the ear'. The ringing sound could also mean that somebody was backbiting the sufferer. A common treatment was to squeeze the juice of an onion into the ear.

**Ear Wax:** Warm a half teaspoonful of olive oil or glycerine and pour into the ear three times a day for two days.

## KIDNEY (INFLAMMATION)

- Apply hot poultices to loins. Eat no food and drink nothing but milk.

## LIVER (SLUGGISH)

People consumed large amounts of honey to draw poisons from the liver (*see* Urine). For any obstruction of liver, bladder or intestines, they pulverised and swallowed dandelion stems.

**Other treatments:**

- Mix two teaspoonfuls of honey in a little water and drink.
- Drink infused hart's-tongue.
- Boil one ounce of chopped dandelion root in one pint of water until it reduces by half. Pulverise horseradish and add a half ounce to the mixture. Stir well and swallow all.

## LUNGS (INFLAMMATION)

- Apply hot oatmeal poultices to the chest and back every four hours.

## OCULAR COMPLAINTS

County Kerry people believed that dabbing eyes with the waters of Tobar na Súl (Eye Well) at Glendahalin, Ballyheigue, could cure mild eye infections or even blindness. A waterfall in Clondaghad, County Clare, is called Saint Screabhan's Well. Screabhan's Bed is close by. Drinking the water and standing in the 'bed' can cure sore eyes. Protection from fairies' wiles is a side benefit!

Other wells promised similar results: Lacken, County Wicklow; Tully, County Galway; Saint Patrick's on the County Leitrim slope of Slieve Anierin; Saint Catherine's, Killybegs, County Donegal (*see also* Holy Wells).

More practical cures included dabbing the eyes

with dampened bread, used tea leaves, dock leaf or oatmeal.

**Other treatments:**

- Boil down petals of daisies and use the liquid as an eyewash.
- Pulverise houseleek and dab its juice on the eyes.
- Dip a plant called *duilleogín Phadraig* ([Saint] Patrick's small leaf) in spring water and bathe.
- Rub on gall from a salmon.
- Rub the eye with a gold wedding band.
- Rub a snail on the eye.
- Mix one teaspoonful of salt to one pint of lukewarm water and bathe each morning and evening. Throughout the day substitute bread soda for salt. Apply a poultice of bread and milk at night.
- Use a teaspoonful of alum to a half pint of water as an eyewash.
- Place a teaspoonful of boric powder in a half cupful of warm water and bathe.
- Close the eye and hold it over the smoke from a burning blessed candle.

**Black Eye:** Mix a teaspoonful of bread soda in a half pint of hot water and bathe.

- Place a wedge of raw meat on the bruise.

**Cataract (*fionn*):** There was a distinction between *fionn* and *fionn ar shúil*, the latter being what was known as a pearl in the eye. Folk cures for both were the same. A macabre example was taking blood from a dead infant and keeping it for rubbing on the eyes as the problems occurred.

**Other treatments:**

- Bathe in a cow's urine.
- Pulverise houseleeks and rub the juice on the eye.
- Apply milk of a nursing mother.

**Removing a Foreign Body from the Eye:** Draw upper lid as far as possible over lower lid.

- One person stands behind the patient and pulls each eyelid open while another removes the foreign body with the corner of a clean cloth.
- Place a drop of castor oil in the eye and roll it about until the foreign body flows out.

**Stye:** Many of the above remedies also cured styes but specific remedies for that affliction included rubbing with a fasting spit, dabbing with dandelion milk and making the Sign of the Cross on the stye with the wedding band of the patient's mother. The most common cure, however, was pointing a thorn or sharp pointed instrument at the stye and calling out *'Imigh! Imigh!'* (Go away! Go away!). Some folk healers stipulated a gooseberry thorn for the ritual.

**Weak Eyes:** Boil daisies, cool and use regularly as eyewash.

- Boil yellow iris in water. When cool, bathe the eyes with the liquid.

FIFTEEN

# RESPIRATORY DISORDERS

'The chest is at me. I'm wheezing like the West Clare at Ennistymon' – in some of their health reports, County Clare people reminded listeners of the gradient overcome by their famous West Clare Railway. In that county, and elsewhere, wearing red flannel across the chest helped many respiratory disorders. Inhaling the steam from boiled concoctions featured also.

## ASTHMA

Centaury, also known as *dréimire Mhuire* (Mary's ladder), appears in folk medicine as a cure for asthma but instructions on its use are vague.

**Other treatments:**

- On the chest place silk that belonged to a mute person who has been dead for seven years.
- Soak red flannel in turpentine and apply to the chest.
- Apply a mustard plaster to the chest.
- Eat watercress.
- Chew coltsfoot.
- Dry mullein leaves. Light them and allow them to smoulder. Inhale the smoke.
- Take the spiny leaves and blue flowers from sea holly. Pulverise, heat and apply to the chest as a poultice.

## BLOCKED SINUSES
Chew beeswax.

## BRONCHITIS
- Chew ivy leaves and swallow the juice.
- Heat comfrey, honey and sugar until it becomes a syrup. Drink while warm.
- Light dried mullein leaves and allow to smoulder. Inhale the smoke.
- Cut a sheet of brown paper in the shape of a heart. Smear with goose grease and apply to chest.
- Take regular mustard baths.
- Pull nine hairs from a black cat. Chop them up and soak them in honey. Swallow some each day.
- Drink the juices from boiled lemons and honey three times a day.
- Mix egg white and linseed oil into a paste. Smear on the chest and on the back and cover with red flannel.

## CATARRH
- Inhale steam of fresh cow's urine.

## COMMON COLD
'Ne'er cast a clout till May is out' applied to adults as well as to children. Men wore long johns (warm underwear) as soon as the first bite of frost came in late autumn. To reinforce their insulation, they

sometimes pinned black paper inside them. (Large black sugar bags were popular and brought a sweet crinkle to their gait!)

'Starve a fever; feed a cold.' Porridge or boiled flaxseed (linseed) was fed to the patient – as much as possible – washed down with beef tea, or porter mulled by immersing a red hot poker in the glass.

At the onset of winter, householders boiled carrageen moss, a fine edible purple seaweed, and allowed it to cool. Drinking it helped cure a cold. Some people added nasturtium seeds.

**Other treatments:**

- A morsel from the breakfast of a man or woman who had the same surname before their marriage could cure a cough – provided they gave it out of charity.
- Sniffing a pine cone helped relieve nasal blockage. Seafarers brought home eucalyptus oil and kept it for treating colds. They sprinkled a few drops on the pillow each night. Inhaling its pleasant aroma helped.
- Honey had a detrimental effect on bacteria and one part diluted in ten of hot water or milk was a simple remedy. This was more effective if the honey was brown and came from poplar trees (*see* Urine).
- If a member of the travelling community caught a cold he threw away the ninth alms received each day.

- Add a fistful each of dandelions, sorrel, hazel buds and groundsel when making oatmeal porridge. Eat a plateful morning and evening.
- Chew mountain sage.
- Drink warm whey.
- Drink donkey's milk.
- Inhale smoke from burning turf.
- Eat boiled turnips.
- Take a mustard bath.
- Chop up and soak nine hairs from a black cat and swallow them.
- Drink the juices from boiled lemons and honey.
- Mix egg white and linseed oil into a paste and smear on the chest.
- Drink hot milk and pepper, with a tiny scrap of butter added (optional extras: porter and sugar).
- Drink a spoonful of any alcohol mixed with sugar and breadcrumbs.
- Best of all (or at least, most popular with the patient!) – drink a few glasses of hot whiskey or *poitín* with cloves or favourite spices and honey. This is called a *scailtín* or, more recently, a hot toddy.

CONGESTION
*See* Pneumonia, *below*.

## CONSUMPTION
*See* Tuberculosis, *below.*

## COUGHING
- Drink camomile tea.
- Bring knobs of butter dipped in sugar to the bedside at night. When a bout of coughing occurs, allow a portion to melt in the mouth and trickle down the throat.
- Gather rosehips. Split them and scrape out the furry seeds. Boil the remainder in a half pint of water until it becomes a syrup. Allow to cool. Mix in the yolk of a fresh egg. Add sugar to taste. Take a few spoonfuls each night before retiring.
- Drink crushed garlic cloves soaked in water until soft.
- Inhale the steam of boiling ivy leaves.
- Mix an egg white with fine sugar and whip to a froth. Take a teaspoonful each hour for four hours.

## FARMER'S LUNG
This is a respiratory disorder resulting from inhaling spores of mouldy hay. To treat, drink flaxseed (linseed) boiled in water.

## HAY FEVER
- Boil one pint of water. Add a teaspoonful of friar's balsam. Inhale the vapour.

- Boil a pinch of pulverised monkshood in a half a pint of milk. Add some *poitín*. Allow to become a whey and take at bedtime.

## HICCUPS

- Give the sufferer a fright.
- Drink water from the opposite side of a glass (difficult, but possible).
- Inhale deeply. Press the nostrils together tightly with the fingers. Hold the breath for as long as possible.

## PLEURISY

Bleeding was regarded as a remedy. At the turn of the twentieth century Michael Forde, a healer from Tullynaha, County Cavan, used a 'flame' (*see* Blood Disorders) to extract a pint from a young male patient. He allowed it to flow into a bowl. Froth began to appear and eventually it covered the surface. Within a week, the patient was cured of pleurisy and lived into his eighties.

**Other treatments:**

- Drink camomile tea.
- Do not eat solids.
- Make poultice of linseed oil and oatmeal or of mustard and apply to the sides.

## PNEUMONIA

- Shear wool from a black sheep. Smear it with fried onions or mustard lubricated with egg white. Apply as a poultice to the chest.

- Rub tallow on the chest. Cover with thick brown paper (black is better, if available).
- Apply a poultice of linseed oil and oatmeal to the chest or back.
- Drink camomile tea.

## SNEEZING

Some local traditions maintained that every sneeze took a second off a lifetime; others, that it could banish the soul from the body. If a person sneezed, therefore, it was customary to say '*Dia duit*' ('God save you') or 'God bless you'. The custom survives.

Incessant sneezing could be an instinctive reaction to the presence of a fairy or evil spirit. It demanded immediate attention.

**Treatments:**
- Inhale camphor or eucalyptus.
- Boil water and pour into a narrow topped jar. Inhale the steam.

## TUBERCULOSIS

Consumption was the common name for pulmonary tuberculosis. There was a great fear of the disease and a saying went: 'March puts the man with consumption in the grave.'

If a person died from this illness, his relatives burned his bed. Taking blood from a stranger by some method was a sinister form of cure. For example, if a relative of a sufferer sought help, he might be told to find a stranger carrying home a catch of rabbits, pay him for one but only take the animal's blood. If the donor had knowledge of this cure, however, he would not oblige, because some relative of his own would 'take' the disease from the recipient's relative.

**Other treatments:**

- Drink one cupful of linseed oil per day. Mixed with honey, it was easier to take.
- Drink a mixture of donkey's milk and porter.
- Have the patient sleep over a cow byre.
- Drink four teaspoons of paraffin oil (kerosene) per day.
- Eat a sandwich of dandelions.
- Emulsify snails in salt. Add sugar and cream and swallow the mixture.
- Pulverise a clove of garlic. Mix into milk and drink.
- Pulverise dandelions, mullein, sage and camomile. Boil and eat when cool.
- Sprinkle salt in a pint of fresh milk each day and drink.
- Drink an egg flip made from two eggs and whiskey.
- Pulverise saffron, lign-aloes and rose stems. Place in rose-water and mix. Soak a linen garment in it and, when dry, wear it.

SIXTEEN

# SKIN

Almost every townland in Ireland had a person who could heal warts and other growths. Some of them still exist. Applying clay on which a donkey's urine had fallen could cure dermal complaints. Mudpacks of bog mud, which was clear of bog-oak chips or pebbles, were useful too and were good for the complexion. Buttermilk and oatmeal packs cured a number of afflictions, including blackheads and rashes. Unfortunate youths who suffered from pimples or boils had to drink the juice of stewed nettles. Sprinkling salt on bed sheets cured hives. Mixing two teaspoonfuls of sulphur in water and drinking it regularly cured itch and a number of skin disorders.

Country people 'raked a fire' at night by placing a sod of turf on the remaining embers in the hearth and covering it with ashes. Next morning they scraped off the ashes and had a small fire ready for stoking. With a heather besom they then swept the hearth clean. Spitting on the clean hearth at this juncture and rubbing that spittle on any skin ailment effected a cure.

## ACNE AND BLACKHEADS

- Hold boiled grass to the face while still hot. Keep there until cold.

- Hold the face over a pot of boiling water.
- Place the hole in the handle of a watch key over the blackhead and press until it pops out. Then apply unsalted butter and sulphur.
- Batter a fistful of groundsel with a beetle. Rub the juice on the pimples.

## BITES

The touch of a seventh son could cure infections from bites and also rabies.

**Other treatments:**

- Kill the animal that bites or scratches and place its fur in the wound. An exception is the rat bite, which calls for killing a weasel and using its skin.
- Clip a hair of the animal that bites into a mixture of pulverised barley and crowfoot. Rub on the wound.
- To prevent hydrophobia (rabies) resulting from the bite of a rabid dog it is necessary to kill the animal, burn it and dispose of the ashes in a stream flowing south.
- Mix two ounces each of treacle and pewter filings with four of garlic and six of rue. Boil in a half gallon of ale and take a large spoonful before breakfast every morning until healed.
- Rub tobacco juice on insect bites.

## BLASTS (FACIAL SWELLINGS)

Pulverise grass, marsh mallow, houseleek and rue. Work into unsalted butter or lard. Fry. Strain off liquid and allow to cool and partially solidify. Use as an ointment.

## BLISTERS

Parents warned children that destroying a bird's nest before the young were hatched out would cause severe blistering. The remedy was a poultice of crab apples.

## BOILS

In all treatments, remove the pus immediately and carefully as it can affect other parts of the skin.

- Point a thorn or sharp pointed instrument at the tip three times, but do not pierce.
- Heat well a bottle whose neck fits around the boil. Place over the boil and press gently. The vacuum formed by the cooling air inside it will draw the pus.
- The *císte uachtair* (cream cake) is a Munster cure. Bake brown flour mixed with cream and brewer's yeast. Dampen and apply to the boil.
- Apply dampened crust of a cowpat.
- Apply a hot poultice of snails collected in the morning dew.
- Apply a hot poultice of wheaten breadcrumbs dampened with boiling water.

- Apply a hot poultice of oatmeal.
- Apply a hot poultice of boiled comfrey roots.
- Apply a hot poultice of cobbler's wax.
- Apply a hot poultice of camomile blooms.
- Apply a hot plaster of rootstock of monkshood (*meacan dáthabha*) that has not been boiled in the patient's home.

BRUISES

- Three times each day, place a red-hot stone into water. Bathe the bruise with the water.
- If a stone causes the bruise, take nine stones, go to a bog hole and immerse the foot in its water. Drop each stone into the water but make sure the ninth stone crosses the immersed foot.
- Apply juice of crushed ivy.
- Paint with white of egg and allow to harden.
- Rub with ends of candles that had lit a wake house.
- Apply the spit of a person who has licked a lizard when young.

BUNIONS

- Apply a poultice of heated tormentil.
- Apply a hot poultice of oatmeal.
- Apply a hot poultice of cobbler's wax.
- Allow a dog to lick the affected part.
- Apply beeswax.
- Pulverise a worm. Heat and apply.

BURNS

- Lick the affected part or allow a dog to lick it.
- Apply bread soda, dry, or mixed into buttermilk. Bandage.
- Apply ground starch or flour thickly to exclude air. Bandage.
- Apply castor oil.
- Apply beeswax.
- Rub gently with the singed fur of a black cat.
- Pulverise a worm. Heat and apply.
- Apply egg yolk mixed with butter. Bandage.
- Paint with white of egg and allow to harden.
- Melt butter. Apply in a plaster.
- Apply a poultice of yellow clay from a limestone quarry.
- Apply juice of crushed ivy.
- Paint with gentian violet.
- Rub with ends of candles that had lit a wake house.
- Apply the spit of a person who has licked a lizard when young.
- Boil sheep's suet and remove tissues. To each pound, add four ounces of beeswax. Warm and stir until blended. Keep in a cool place and apply when needed. Bandages dipped in the mixture and allowed to harden may be stored for fast application.
- Mix fresh goose excrement, camomile petals and newly churned, unsalted butter.

- Bathe in urine of a horse or cow.
- Apply a poultice of warm cow dung.
- Apply a hot poultice of pulverised cabbage leaves.
- For one month, allow a dead crane (heron) to decompose in a keg buried in a manure heap. Pour off the remaining liquid and retain for treating burns.
- Boil sheep's suet with elder bark. Mix it into an ointment and apply when cool. This will heal a burn without leaving a scar.
- Pound ivy or dandelion leaves. Rub the juice on the affected area. This cures scalds, burns, abrasions and even ulcers.
- For lime burns, bathe with a mixture of water and vinegar. Grind chalk into linseed oil until it forms a paste. Apply at hourly intervals.

## CARBUNCLES
- Bathe with a cow's urine.

(All entries under Boils [above] also apply to carbuncles.)

## CHAPPED LIPS OR LIP BLISTERS (COLD SORES)
- Write the patient's name with black ink above or below the mouth.
- Hold an ivy leaf between the lips for as long as possible.

- Kill a mouse (people believed the ailment was caused by a mouse's urine. Seeing a sufferer, they remarked, 'I see the mouse pissed on you!').

## CHAPPED SKIN
- Bathe with a cow's urine.
- Apply castor oil.
- Lick the affected part or allow a dog to lick it.

## CHICKEN POX
- Burn rushes and allow the ashes to cool. Add a pinch of gunpowder. Blend into rendered hog's fat and use as an ointment.

## CHILBLAINS
- An early twentieth-century cure suggested that 'a 14% solution of tannic acid, resorcin and ichthyol in water, painted on the affected parts daily will eventually cure the worst cases of chilblains within a week'.

**Other treatments:**
- Pass one's own urine on the affected area or immerse the feet in a basin of it for a half hour.
- Bake a turnip in a pot-oven. Remove skin and mash. Mix in linseed oil and mustard and use as a poultice.
- Dab with forge water or olive oil.

footed in soft bog that covers the
\_\_ fifteen minutes each day for three
weeks. The feet should be pushed through the
bog rather than taking steps. All turns should
be taken to the left, not to the right.

- Dissolve washing soda in tepid water and soak
  for thirty minutes.
- Place a fistful of ivy in a pint of vinegar.
  Bottle, cork tightly and allow it to stand for
  two days. Remove ivy and dab the liquid on
  the corn.
- Tie a heated ivy leaf around the corn.
- Tie a heated houseleek around the corn.
- Pare with a sharp knife or razor.
- Apply beeswax.
- Apply a hot poultice of cobbler's wax.
- Pulverise a worm. Heat and apply.

CYST
- Touch with the hand of a corpse.

DANDRUFF
*See* Head.

ECZEMA
- Mix in a pinch of red oxide of mercury with
  one ounce of lard. Use as an ointment.
- Drink copious amounts of buttermilk.

- Clean a fistful of watercress. Cover with water in a pot and boil. Strain. Cool the liquid and use for bathing the affected area.
- Drink goat's milk.

### ERYSIPELAS

This acute contagious inflammation is accompanied by violent headache, fever and spreading red patches on the skin. Folk medicine erroneously called it Saint Anthony's Fire (*see below*).

### FRECKLES

Freckles were regarded as attractive in a young girl but some parents wished to remove them.

**Treatments:**

- Wash in dew gathered at dawn on May Day (1 May).
- Pulverise horseradish and steep in sour milk for four hours. Wash the face in the mixture each night and morning.
- Overnight, steep hazelnuts or walnuts in the blood of a hare or a bull and wash the face in it regularly.
- Drink distilled water in which hazelnuts or walnuts have been soaked.

### HEAD LICE

Head lice and their eggs (nits) were once a major problem, particularly in children. Night after night, distraught mothers washed and fine-tooth-combed children's hair, the nits dropping onto a sheet of paper on a table. They killed them individually by pressing the thumbnail against them. Severe cases required shaving the head, burning the hair and washing the scalp. Parents then removed any crusts formed by soaking them in olive oil before bedtime and washing next morning. This continued for a week. After each wash, they rubbed sulphur ointment into the scalp.

**Other treatments:**

- Rub paraffin oil on the head to kill the lice.
- To destroy nits, mix four tablespoons of water with one of vinegar and rub vigorously into the scalp. Then part the hair in a number of areas with the fingers, pick out the nits and kill them.

HEAD SCRUFF

Dip a strip of flannel in olive oil and rub the head gently with it. This will soften the scruff. Wash well. Rub in an ointment of sulphur and lard.

**Inflammation**

- Dry nine handfuls of moss from a mountain until it becomes a powder. Each Tuesday and Thursday, mix nine pinches of it with nine of ashes, and swallow.
- Chew dandelion stems.

### ITCH

- Strip and place all the patient's clothes in a pot-oven and heat them for one hour.
- Rub in an ointment of sulphur and lard at night. Wash next morning.
- Rub on an equal mixture of linseed oil and limewater.
- Mix two teaspoonfuls of sulphur in water and drink.

### LEPROSY

Drinking the waters of a spa at Swanlinbar, County Cavan, could cure this dreaded ailment.

### LICE

Body lice only affect areas covered by clothes. Sores may develop on affected parts.

**Treatments:**

- Bathe in warm water and cover the body with pulverised ragwort mixed in linseed oil.
- Paraffin oil will kill crab lice but not their eggs. Treat the general condition by making an ointment of sulphur, the contents of a blue bag and some butter. Rub in well at night and bathe the next morning.

  (*See also* Head Lice, *above*.)

### NODE

- Spread on the white of an egg and allow to harden.

- Apply a poultice of foxglove.

## RABIES
*See* Bites, *above*.

## RASH
- Rubbing a raw garlic clove over the affected areas cures a mild rash.
- A prayer said over a person with severe rash went:

  What will heal thee from the red, thirsty, shivering disease of the foreigner that kills with poisonous pain? The prayer of Mary to her Son and of Columcille to God will.

Another prayer was often said:

  Mary, Patrick, Brigid and Solomon banish from you this redness.

## ROSACEA (ROSE)
- At midnight, remove mud from the boggy base of Lough Leighis (the Healing Lake) near Bailieborough, County Cavan. Use as a mudpack on the affected part.

## SAINT·ANTHONY'S FIRE (ERGOTISM)
Sanit Anthony's fire was a crippling disease, resulting from ergot poisoning. While it often caused

miscarriage and other female problems, it was noted mainly for its gangrenous nature, itching skin and numbness. During the eleventh century, tramps suffering from ergotism were unwanted and despised, and roamed Europe in large groups. In 1093, a son of Gaston de Dauphiné recovered from the disease. In thanksgiving, his father inaugurated the Hospital Brothers of Saint Anthony at Isenheim, Alsace, to house and attend to the wandering sufferers. The name Saint Anthony's Fire for the ailment may have originated from that story.

One old treatment required a male healer to whisper a secret supplication over a slab of butter. He then rubbed the butter on the affected parts of a female patient. A female healer performed a similar procedure for a male patient. The most common cure, however, was applying the blood of a male Keogh to the affected areas. Blood of other families was less effective but could be substituted if a Keogh were not available. These included Cahills, Geoghans, Goughs and Walshes.

**Others treatments:**

- With the index finger, a person with the same surname as the patient traces the patient's surname around the affected part.
- Apply a cow-dung poultice.
- Scald some flour with boiling water and apply.
- Apply paint to the affected area and allow to dry. When the paint eventually cracks and disintegrates, the ailment will be cured.

## SCALDS

- Apply juice of crushed ivy (*see* Burns, *above*).
- Collect a bucket of the first snow of winter. Thaw, bottle and keep for rubbing on scalds.

## SCURVY

Weakness, softening of the gums and particularly haemorrhages under the skin are symptoms of scurvy. Seamen on long voyages and deprived of Vitamin C suffered from it. Lord Nelson attempted to combat it by issuing a daily ration of lime fruit to his sailors, which led to Americans calling British seamen 'limeys'.

Boatmen carried people suffering from scurvy from Coliemore Harbour to Dalkey Island (formerly Torn Island, from the Norse) in Dublin Bay, where drinking the water of Saint Begnet's Well (also Benedict), there helped their ailments.

**Other treatments:**

- Bathe in a stream that touches three mearings.
- Drink waters from a spa near Wexford town (*see* Jaundice, *under* Blood Disorders).
- Mix some sulphur into newly churned butter. Place in mouth and allow to melt and trickle down the throat.

## SHINGLES

- Rub on the blood of a Cahill.
- Apply a fasting spit and make the Sign of the Cross with a wedding band.

- Apply zinc ointment.
- Apply zinc oxide and powdered starch.

## SKIN CANCER
*See* Cancer.

## SKIN CARE
- Apply mudpack of bog mud.
- Wash the skin in fresh human urine.
- Soak oatmeal in water. Use as a face pack or thin out more and use as a lotion.
- Regularly wash the face in buttermilk.
- Cut a cucumber and rub the inside over the skin.
- Rub in juice from comfrey root.

## SMALLPOX
Isolate the patient and put to bed. Sponge and apply a mixture of linseed and limewater.

## SORES
- Boil foxglove. Sweeten with honey. Allow to cool. Drink it or rub it on the affected part.
- Make an ointment from rendered beef suet and yarrow and apply.
- Roast chickweed in a pot-oven and place on the sore.
- Pulverise ragwort (*buachalán buí*). Heat and apply as a poultice.

- Apply an ointment made from goose grease and crushed tansy.
- Boil dock roots. Cool and drink.
- Apply juice from pulverised dock leaves.
- For sores on the soles of feet, place stewed sorrel in the patient's boots or shoes and wear without stockings.

  (*See also* Ulcers, *below*.)

## SPLINTER REMOVAL

Pulverise a tiny portion of resin. Place on a piece of linen. Drop hot tallow grease on the resin and apply to the affected area to draw out the splinter. Treatments for removing thorns also apply.

## STINGS

**Nettle stings:** Rub spittle on a dock leaf and apply, saying:

> *Chuir an neantóg cealg ionnam;*
> *Copóg shráide mo leigheas.*
> [A] nettle stung me;
> [A] dock cured me.

- Rub with rosemary or mint leaves.

**Jellyfish stings:**

- Urinate on the sting. (Recently, doctors have warned against this traditional cure. They say it merely cools the skin, giving temporary relief

to something that could cause a severe allergic
reaction, leading to breathing difficulties and,
in extreme cases, death.)

**Bee (or wasp) stings:**

- Rub with a damp blue bag.
- Cut an onion and rub the inside on the sting.
- Apply cow dung.
- Squeeze out the sting by pressing the hole in
  the handle of a watch key around the location,
  then dab with vinegar or bread soda in water.

## SUNBURN

- Soak two teaspoonfuls of quince seed in a
  teacupful of cold water for two days. Apply to
  affected area.
- Mix half a teaspoonful of bread soda with two
  tablespoonfuls each of water and glycerine.
  Wash the affected area with the preparation.
- Apply cream, unsalted butter or a mixture of
  buttermilk and bread soda.

## SWELLINGS

- Make a poultice from crushed daffodil stalks
  and apply.
- Pulverise chickweed and elm bark. Steep for
  one hour and apply in a plaster.
- Touch the affected part with nine different
  irons (poker, tongs, etc.) three times on a
  Tuesday or Thursday, while praying.

### THRUSH (ORAL)

- Put the beak of a fasting gander in the patient's mouth.
- Press breath from a dead child onto the patient's mouth.
- Drop milk left by an infant that died into the patient's mouth.
- Have a 'left twin' (survivor of twins when one dies) breathe in the patient's mouth three times.
- Chew plantain.
- Pulverise gentian blooms and paint the infected area with the juice. Keep the mouth open until it dries.
- Have a man born after his father died breathe into the patient's mouth three times.
- Chew the under part of a rusting dock leaf.

### ULCERS

Some homes kept placentas of cows and even humans for treatment of ulcers or deep sores. They dried them in the chimney and applied a portion to the ulcer, keeping it in place with a bandage.

**Other treatments:**

- Boil a ray until jellied. Remove bones. Apply and bandage.
- Apply leaves of ragwort and figwort. Bandage.
- Apply a poultice of dock leaves, cabbage leaves, dandelions or cow dung.

- Mix the blood of a Keogh with newly churned, unsalted butter. Apply and bandage.

## WARTS

Many still go to people who have 'the cure' for warts. In some cases, a visit is not necessary. As long as the healer knows the name of the patient, he can cure from a distance. DIY wart removers, however, were common, even in the recent past. Many cures demanded treatment at dawn on one Thursday and two Mondays. Cutting off the blood supply by tying a horse's hair around the base of the wart could succeed if the base was narrow.

If a man who had licked a 'laca leech' also licked a wart, it would disappear within days. (A 'laca leech' is a hard-skinned creature about two inches long and a half inch thick. It clings to stones in streams.)

**Other treatments:**

- Cauterise the wart with a red hot needle or by careful application of caustic soda, sulphuric or nitric acid.
- Cut a potato, rub the inner surface of one half on the wart, and then bury it. Repeat the procedure the following day with the second half. The wart will disappear as the potato rots.
- Tie as many knots on a string of wool as the patient has warts. Bury the wool.
- Cut as many notches in an elder branch as the patient has warts.

- Pick as many alder shoots as the number of warts on the patient. Bury the shoots.
- Make the Sign of the Cross on the wart with an elder leaf.
- Without his knowing it, touch a garment on a man who never knew his father.
- Apply fasting spittle each morning until the wart disappears.
- Dab on dandelion milk each morning until the wart disappears.
- Dab on milk from milkwort or spurge daily.
- Touch each wart with a pebble and leave the stones in a pile at a crossroads. The person who knocks over the pile will take the warts from the patient.
- Apply some earth from the sole of a boot of a man bearing a coffin and ask the wart to disappear.
- Attend a funeral. Stroke the wart with a needle in the direction in which the cortège is moving and say, 'Dead man, dead! Take my wart with you.'
- Sew a few pebbles and a silver coin in a pouch. Leave on a road. Whoever finds the bag and keeps the money will also take the warts from the patient.
- Apply calf dung mixed with vinegar.
- Apply goat's droppings mixed with unsalted butter or vinegar.
- Apply a stolen scrap of raw meat. Bury it in

the ground. The wart will decay as the meat decays. Nobody must observe the theft or the burial.

- Apply a stolen scrap of raw meat. Leave it in a place where it will be found easily. The person who takes it will also take the warts.
- Apply a mixture of rendered beef fat and rue.
- Place a stone in a pot for boiling potatoes. When potatoes boil, take out the stone and rub the wart with it.
- Rub with any stone.
- Rub with juice of spurge.
- Rub with a dirty tea towel while calling: *'Imigh! Imigh! Imigh!'* (Away! Away! Away!). Bury the towel in the light of a full moon.
- Point a thorn or pin at the wart and call 'Away! Away! Away!' then place the pin in water and as it rusts, the wart will disappear.
- Apply castor oil daily for one week.
- Rub with bacon fat and bury the fat.
- Apply forge water at dawn for nine mornings and leave the container where somebody might steal it. If that happens, the wart will disappear.
- Bathe with water from boiled potatoes.
- Bathe with froth from a fast-running stream.
- Take some water from a hollow in a stone discovered by accident. Rub it on the wart three times, saying each time:

*Uisce cloiche gan iarraidh! Ní dhot' iarraidh*
*atá mé. Bhíos ag dul abhaile agus casadh*
*liom thú.*

Water of unsought stones, I was not
looking for you. I was going home and
met you.

(*See also* Holy Wells.)

WHITLOW (WHITTLE)
- Apply water from boiling potatoes.
- Apply a poultice of spurge.
- Apply a poultice of grass, yarrow, bog cotton
  (*ceannbhán*) and egg white. Leave for two days.
- The cures for Blasts and Warts (*above*) also
  cure whitlows.

WINDBURN
- Clean a fistful of watercress. Cover with water
  in a pot and boil. Strain. Dab the affected area
  with the cress. Cool the liquid and use later for
  washing the affected area.

SEVENTEEN

# STOMACH AND BOWELS

## STOMACH

What country people referred to as a 'bad stomach' was very often the upper abdominal pain associated with a duodenal ulcer. There was no definite folk remedy for this complaint but some patients took treacle, raw eggs in milk, clear soup and chicken broth. Apart from chicken, they avoided all other fowl. Their diet often consisted of black tea and bread toasted on one side only. Chronic cases visited Teach Dorcha (Dark House), a ruin in a cemetery in Kilbarry, County Roscommon. Under its entrance, allegedly, was the grave of Saint Barry. The patient took clay from there and rubbed it on his stomach. Similar treatment cured headaches and other ailments.

Healers often concluded that ailments came from an evil presence. The belief that abnormal hunger resulted from ingesting an *earc luachra* (rush lizard) is an example. The treatment was comic. The healer tied the sufferer's feet to the rafters and placed a plate of currant cake or some sweet-smelling dish below his mouth to coax out the lizard. Worse, he might give the patient some disgusting concoction to eat or drink to force out the intruder.

Irish folk-medicine practitioners called the sword-shaped (ensiform) cartilage at the base of the breastbone the *cléithín* and used the word to describe the feeling of indigestion that occurs when the 'breastbone is down'. They cured it by pressing a warmed glass over the cartilage area. The contracting air inside lifted it into its proper place. Sometimes they placed oatmeal dough on the spot, stuck a lit candle in it and covered it with a glass. This created a better vacuum. *Poitín* or whiskey and port were popular remedies for an 'unsettled stomach' and many malingerers pleaded for the cure.

### Biliousness

*   Drink waters from a spa near Wexford town (*see* Jaundice, *under* Blood Disorders).

### Colic

*   Chew mountain sage.
*   Heat red flannel and apply to stomach.
*   Make a poultice of hot bran and apply to stomach.
*   Boil a lemon in water. Add pepper and drink.
*   Relieve bowels (*see* Constipation, *below*).

### Heartburn (Heart Fever)

*   A healer prayed while holding a cupful of oatmeal in his hand. If his prayers were heard,

a hollow would form in the oatmeal. The patient took the meal, baked a cake using it and ate it throughout the following morning.

**Other treatments:**

- Lick the back of a lizard.
- Mix a teaspoonful of bread soda into a half pint of water and drink.

## *Indigestion*

For severe indigestion, useful emetics consisted of (a) a half tablespoonful of mustard in a cupful of hot water, or (b) four tablespoonfuls of sea salt in a glass of lukewarm water.

**Other treatments:**

- Drink a pint of water last thing at night and first thing in the morning. If severe, add bread soda.
- Swallow ten dandelion stems.
- Chew mountain sage.
- Pulverise columbine and gentian. Add a teaspoonful of bread soda. Infuse and drink three tablespoonfuls daily before the main meal.
- Take the juice of one lemon after each meal.

## *Stomach Ache*

- Drink thyme, marjoram or camomile tea.
- Tie a sprig of mint around the wrist.
- Mix soot in water and drink.

- Chew raw garlic.
- Heat comfrey, honey and sugar until it becomes a syrup. Drink while warm.
- Pass through a *Crios Bhríde* or tie it around the stomach (*see* Protection from Evil and Sickness).

### Summer Fever

- Follow the instructions for Indigestion, *above*.

### Vomiting

- Drink thyme tea.

## BOWELS

### Constipation

Before laxatives like castor oil, Epsom Salts, Kruschen Salts or fruit pastilles became available, people drank tea made from senna pods (from cassia, or cheap cinnamon). Earlier still, eating onions or chewing raw garlic cloves kept the bowels in order.

A doctor once told me how he had prescribed castor oil for a woman suffering from constipation. She misunderstood and drank paraffin oil (kerosene). After returning in severe pain, the conversation went something like this:

Doctor: Did you take the castor oil?

Woman: Jaysus, Doctor, I thought you said paraffin oil. Oh Lord! What will I do?

Doctor: Stick a wick up your arse and you'll have light for the winter.

**Other treatments:**

- Drink a pint of warm water before breakfast.
- Boil onions in milk. Eat the onions and drink the milk, preferably at bedtime.
- Drink castor oil (in mutton broth, water and brandy or hot milk to disguise the taste).
- Chew aloes.
- Insert soap in the anus.

*Diarrhoea*

- Drink the milky juice of mountain spurge (*meacan buí an tsléibhe*; lit. yellow root of the mountain).
- Beat the whites of two eggs and add to a pint of water in which two teaspoonfuls of salt have dissolved. Take a fifth of the mixture immediately. Vomiting should occur inside fifteen minutes. If not, take the remainder. Repeat the dose four times daily, if necessary.
- Boil roots or buds of the blackberry bramble in a little water and drink while warm.
- Boil yellow iris in water. Drink while warm.
- Seafarers sometimes brought home pomegranates. They squeezed out the juice from one, added sugar and drank it. Sometimes they used an Arabian cure that involved drying the skin of the fruit, infusing

it and drinking the concoction. Steeping the fruit and drinking the water was another method. This treatment also helped dysentery.

### Dysentery

- Pulverise some maidenhair fern and woodbine blossom. Mix with oatmeal and boil in new milk. Take three times each day. When cured, burn any of the mixture that remains.
- Heat comfrey, honey and sugar until it becomes a syrup. Drink while warm.
- Beat one egg. Mix in some sugar. Drink the concoction three times each day until cured. Place any hot poultice on the stomach to relieve pain. (*See* Diarrhoea, *above*.)

### Flatulence

- Dissolve two teaspoonfuls of bread soda in a glass of water and drink.
- Mix four teaspoonfuls of soot into a half pint of fresh milk and drink.

EIGHTEEN

# TEETH

Too many country people neglected their teeth dreadfully. A local 'tooth man', often the blacksmith, pulled out teeth with catgut or strong thread. He threw dislodged teeth over the right shoulder and never looked at them again.

Hart's-tongue was applied to sore or bleeding gums or after tooth removal.

Sometimes a man suffering from toothache went to a cemetery and prayed over a grave for the repose of the soul of the person buried there. Then he pulled a few blades of grass from the grave and chewed it well before spitting it out. The pain left with the discharge. Promising Jesus, Mary and a new moon that he would never comb his hair on a Friday could help too. The trouble was, however, that thereafter he had to fall on his knees and pray every time he saw a full moon – even if he happened to be wading through water.

Some people believed that a worm in the tooth caused toothache. They had a prayer pleading for its destruction.

Not shaving on a Sunday kept a toothache away, as did wearing a 'gospel' with the verse:

Saint Peter was sitting, all alone,
Beside the Lord on his marble throne,
Who asked, 'Oh, Peter, what makes you shake?'
'My Lord it is this severe toothache.'
The Lord said, 'Wear this for My sake
And never more will you have a toothache.'

**Other treatments:**

- Rub the affected tooth with a molar extracted from a skull unearthed on Hallowe'en.
- The patient pulls the tooth from a skeleton with his own teeth.
- Chew the root of ragwort.
- Rub the tooth of a dead horse over the jawbone.
- Recite the Lord's Prayer, and follow by saying aloud: 'May the hand of Thomas in Christ's wound rid my tooth of worms and pain.'
- Chew cloves or freshly pulled yarrow.
- Drink a mixture of alum and vinegar.
- Touch the nerve with a horseshoe nail.
- Pour a drop of *poitín* or whiskey into the cavity.
- Pack a wad of plug tobacco or clay from an elder root in the cavity.
- Put some bluestone in the cavity.
- Rub a live frog on the tooth.
- Rub mustard on the gums.

NINETEEN

# THROAT

The Irish used the word 'craw' for the 'throat'. If a person said 'It stuck in my craw', he had heard something that was difficult to accept. A crawthumper was a hypocrite (who beat his breast in prayer) and being crawsick was to suffer from a hangover.

Candlemas Day falls on 2 February and candles blessed on that day were used the following day, the feast day of Saint Blaise, for the blessing of throats. A priest uttered a specified prayer while holding two crossed candles before the recipient's neck. Although Blaise (died *c.* 316) was an Armenian wool-comber, devotion to him was popular in Ireland, particularly among livestock farmers. They believed that praying to him, especially on his feast day, could cure ailing cattle.

## GOITRE

- Touch the throat with the hand of a corpse.

## LARYNGITIS

- Rest the voice, do not smoke and use the treatments for bronchitis (*see* Respiratory Disorders).

## MUMPS

- Rubbing the patient's head against a pig's back cured mumps – but the pig got the malady!

**Other treatments:**

- Ask advice from a man riding a white horse.
- Bring the patient to a mearing where three townlands meet.
- Before dawn, gather nine black stones, preferably from a stream. After bringing the patient to a holy well in silence, throw away the stones, one by one. While casting each of the first three, say 'In the name of God'. Follow with 'In the name of Christ' for the second three, and 'In the name of Mary' for the final three. Do this on each of three mornings.
- Place a donkey's halter on the patient and lead him to a river flowing south. The patient then drinks the water directly, without using any utensil.
- Place a donkey's halter on the patient and lead him three times around a pigsty.
  (*See also* Whooping Cough, *under* Children.)

## SORE THROAT

- Gargle with salted water.
- Pulverise seaweed. Dip the tip of a narrow twig in it and paint the back of the throat through the mouth (when iodine became available, it was substituted for the seaweed juice).

- Mix a half teaspoonful each of alum and sulphuric acid with two teaspoonfuls of treacle. Dissolve in a half pint of warm water and gargle.
- Apply a poultice of boiled bay leaf.
- Heat sea salt and place in a stocking. Wear around the neck like a scarf.
- Mix a half pint of turpentine with two raw eggs. Pour into a two-pint, lidded, container and shake vigorously until creamy. Add one pint of vinegar, one tablespoonful of ammonia and a camphor ball. Use as an embrocation. (The preparation will last for years.)
- Allow honey to trickle down the throat.
- Chew elderberries.
- Massage with goose droppings.
- Chew a garlic bulb.
- Ingest self-heal (a variety of prunella) by any method.
- Drink hot milk and pepper, mixed with a little butter, porter and sugar.

TONSILITIS
- Tug the hair on the top of the head repeatedly.
- Gargle with salted water.
- Inhale steam from two ounces of friar's balsam boiled in a pint of water.
- Crush a garlic clove and mix with honey. Allow to trickle down the throat.
- Place hot potatoes or sea salt in a woollen

stocking. Wrap around the throat. (In later years, a caterpillar or 'hairy molly' [butterfly larva] in a lisle or silk stocking was substituted.)

- Rub the head and neck with a freshly roasted potato.

    (*See also* Ribín Bhríde, *in* Headaches and Migraine, *under* Head.)

TWENTY

# URINE

In times past, people were reticent about mentioning any urinary complaint. They often suffered in silence and even died without treatment. Sometimes they whispered about *an galar fuail* (the blood disease). A pagan charm called on birds and witches to help and was displayed in whatever place served as a lavatory. Although they referred to 'stones' and 'gravel', folk practitioners did not have precise definitions in the case of kidney stones, gall stones and other complaints, and they massaged the area of pain or of difficulty with a fox's blood. For example, an enlarged prostate gland presented problems passing water especially in older men but this was understood by only a few healers.

Householders used honey in many treatments but especially for urinary problems. They knew the type of honey that came from certain plants and suggested remedies accordingly. Brown honey came from poplar trees, green from thistles, white from fireweed and yellow from golden rod. Their confidence was supported by Doctor W.B. Schwasheimer who wrote in *New Health* in 1938: 'Honey [is excellent] for suppuration of the bladder and nephritis because it stimulates the activities of the kidneys and intestines.'

Chewing parsley and dandelions or drinking 'dandelion tea' helped too (the name 'piss-a-bed' for a dandelion survives). Eating cranesbill, a variety of geranium, or sucking the juice of juniper berries assisted the flow of urine, as did drinking copious amounts of spring water.

## BRIGHT'S DISEASE (BRIOS BRÚN)
An acute or chronic inflammation of the kidneys (nephritis).
**Treatments:**
- Eat the joints from the redshank, a large sandpiper (*glúineach dhearg*).

## DIABETES
*See* Blood Disorders.

## GRAVEL
*Tinneas uisce,* lit. 'water sickness'. Sandy substance in urine that, if congealed, could form a stone (*see* Stones, *below*).
**Treatments:**
- Chew mouse-ear hawkweed (*cluas liath*).
- Chew bilberry (*fraochán*, whortleberry) leaves.
- Boil pearl barley in water and drink copious amounts.
- Eat raw onions.
- Boil barley grain in water. Allow to cool and drink frequently.
- Apply poultices to the stomach and loins to relieve pain.

## INCONTINENCE

- Drink the juice of pulverised turnips to control urine.

## KIDNEYS

- Drink at least a half gallon of water each day.
- Chew bilberry leaves in the spring and summer and its fruit in autumn.
- Squeeze cranberries and drink the juice.

## PROSTATE GLAND

For difficulty passing urine, boil four tablespoonfuls of pearl barley in four pints of water and drink each day.

## STONES

- In three pints of water, boil four fistfuls each of bog cotton (*ceannbhán*) heads and pellitory-of-the-wall (*miontas caisil*, a low, green-flowering bushy plant found at bases of walls). After three hours, strain and bottle. Swallow or mix with heated oatmeal and use as a poultice on the region of the bladder.
- Boil roots of butcher's broom (a low, spiny evergreen) in two pints of water. Add one pint of whiskey or *poitín* and honey to taste. Strain and store in bottles. Take three glasses daily.
- Boil two ounces of pearl barley in one and a half pints of water. Strain and drink the liquid.

# GLOSSARY

**antiphlogistine:** A veterinary product that allays
   inflammation; from the noun antiphlogistic.

**archangel tar:** A preparation manufactured from
   the residue after turpentine has been distilled
   from coniferous wood, normally pine.

**bread soda:** sodium bicarbonate

*cáise Púca:* (cosha Pooka. Lit. Pooka's cheese.
   Puffball) a round-shaped fungus filled with
   brown powder found in a field.

**conach worm/moth:** Conach worm – the
   caterpillar of the elephant hawk moth. Conach
   moth – the elephant hawk moth.

*crios:* belt

**crubeen:** pig's trotter

**Daithini:** a Munster faction

**dulse:** (*dileasg*) an edible seaweed

**elf-stone:** Fairy stone, usually a Stone Age
   arrowhead, found in or near a fairy rath. Once
   dug out, it should never again touch the
   ground, or its power would disappear.

**Fionn Mac Cumhaill:** Leader of the Fianna who were
   bodyguards of the High King. Fionn was one of
   the most renowned warriors in Irish mythology.

**fuller's earth:** A clay-like substance normally used
   to clean or add body to cloth. It acts as a
   catalyst in some chemical reactions.

**Gearaltaigh:** a Munster faction

**gospel:** A small card containing a prayer worn on the person, often on a string around the neck, or sewn in a garment.

**mearing:** boundary fence or ditch separating two farms

**O'Neill, Hugh:** Third Baron Dungannon and Second Earl of Tyrone (1550–1616). A flamboyant warrior.

*piseóg*(a): Superstition(s). Charm or old wives' tale. Also pishogue or pishrogue.

*poitín:* (poteen) Illicit spirits made from potatoes. Mountain dew.

**slash-hook:** straight or slightly hooked blade on a handle used for cutting thick hedges